"Esther Gokhale's vision of what makes a healthy back will be startling to most Americans, because it is so different from what we have always learned. But if we just give it a chance, her vision will become ours, with the clarity of something that seems obvious once it is pointed out. With the adoption of even a few of Esther's precepts, a life of bad habits can change to a life of healthy sitting and moving, and therefore a life of less pain and more freedom. The Gokhale Method℠ is, for most of us, a new way of looking at and taking care of our backs, but for those of us who have read this book or learned about it in person, it will become the only way."

— **Jessica Davidson**, M.D., Internal Medicine, Palo Alto Medical Foundation, CA

"This is an amazing book, documenting the writer's unique expertise and a truly visionary approach to myofascial back pain. Back problems are not only pervasive, but also intractable and expensive, frequently disabling, commonly resulting in overmedication and unnecessary surgery that only aggravates the pain and leads to more disability. *8 Steps to a Pain-Free Back* is comprehensive yet written in concise, easy-to-comprehend language. The illustrations are excellent and provide a self-explanatory course of treatment; thoughtful anthropological asides are both entertaining and insightful. This book and the therapeutic approach it documents are great assets to all of us who deal with back pain daily in our practices: neurologists, physical therapists, physiatrists, general practitioners, and of course, to the patients themselves."

— **Helen Barkan**, M.D., Ph.D., Neurology, Mayo Clinic, Rochester, MN

"In six 1-hour sessions I felt transformed. The approach is stunningly simple and confers immediate results. I wholeheartedly endorse this program."

— **Deirdre Stegman**, M.D., Palo Alto Medical Foundation, CA

"I see tons of 'slouching and tucking' in my Pediatric office and a surprising number of children and teens with back pain. I have been referring many of my patients to Esther and will be recommending this book routinely."

— **Tina McAdoo**, M.D., Pediatrics, Palo Alto Medical Clinic, CA

"The fresh and thoughtful approach to preventing and treating back pain presented by Esther Gokhale in this book deserves the attention of the medical profession. We have not served our patients with back pain well, and the techniques so well-described in this book hold the promise of significant relief to a very common and distressing problem."

— **Harvey J. Cohen**, MD, PhD, Professor of Pediatrics, Stanford University School of Medicine, CA

"Back pain is one of the most common problems seen in primary care. Unfortunately, many patients and clinicians are frustrated by the limitations of medical or surgical therapy in providing sustained relief for what is often a recurrent or chronic problem. Esther Gokhale has produced a clearly written, beautifully illustrated book which presents an extensively researched, carefully refined, natural approach to treating and preventing back pain. In this book, patients will find an integrated set of exercises and posture techniques designed to provide long term relief for their pain. Clinicians will find information on exercises and posture training they can use to help their patients who suffer from back pain."

— **David Thom**, M.D., Ph.D., Professor of Family and Community Medicine, University of California, San Francisco, CA

Remember When It Didn't Hurt

8 STEPS to a
PAIN-FREE
BACK

*Natural posture solutions for pain in the back,
neck, shoulder, hip, knee, and foot*

ESTHER GOKHALE, L.Ac.
WITH SUSAN ADAMS

 Pendo Press

To the millions of people who suffer needlessly from back pain

8 Steps to a Pain-Free Back.
Natural posture solutions for pain in the back, neck,
shoulder, hip, knee, and foot.

This book is printed on acid-free paper.

Printed and bound in China.

Publisher's Cataloging-in-Publication
(Provided by Quality Books, Inc.)

Gokhale, Esther.
    8 steps to a pain-free back : natural posture
  solutions for pain in the back, neck, shoulder, hip,
  knee, and foot / Esther Gokhale ; with Susan Adams.
      p. cm. -- (Remember when it didn't hurt)
    Includes bibliographical references and index.
    LCCN 2007937362
    ISBN-13: 978-0-9793036-0-9
    ISBN-10: 0-9793036-0-5

    1. Back--Care and hygiene. 2. Backache--Treatment.
  3. Posture.   I. Adams, Susan, 1944- II. Title.
  III. Title: Eight steps to a pain-free back. IV. Series.

  RD771.B217G65 2008   617.5'64
                        QBI07-600232

Attention: Quantity discounts are available for corporations,
medical groups, retirement homes, educational institutions,
and sports organizations for resale, teaching, subscription
incentives, gifts, or fund raising. Organizations interested in
specialized books or excerpts: please contact Special Sales,
Pendo Press, 2439 Birch Street, Suite 1, Palo Alto, CA
94306. Phone 1-888-557-6788. Fax: 1-650-327-1603.
Email: info@gokhalemethod.com.

ACKNOWLEDGMENTS

Many, many people helped make this book happen—friends, colleagues, teachers, subjects, patients, students, and family. In particular, I would like to thank:

My parents, Manohar Krishna Gokhale and Wilma Meijer, who gave me my first lessons in navigating multiple cultures and gleaning the best from them.

Noelle Perez-Christiaens, for pioneering the field of anthropologically-informed posture and movement work. Noelle is the first person I know to identify the importance of pelvic anteversion, and to recommend lengthening the spine for extended periods. What I learned from her is the foundation of much of what I present in this book.

B.K.S. Iyengar (yoga), Elly Vunderink-de Vries (yoga), Kutti Krishnan (Bharata Natyam), Georgia Leconte (Aplomb), Alain Girard (Aplomb), Angelika Thusius (Kentro), Karen Mattison (Pilates), Regine N'Dounda (Congolese dance), Wilfred Mark (Caribbean dance), Benny Duarte (Brazilian dance), Marsea Marquis (Brazilian dance), Beiçola (Capoiera, Brazilian dance), Dandha da Hora (Brazilian dance), and Massengo (Congolese drumming), for contributing to my work with techniques, understanding, or inspiration.

Susan Adams, for volunteering 18 months of invaluable help clarifying and polishing the text. Her remarkable stamina, perseverance, and linguistic skill kept the project in motion till the finish.

Gaith Kawar, for his patient instruction in InDesign at the Palo Alto Apple Store, followed by his expertise as the book's layout designer.

Brett Miller, for drawing and redrawing almost all the illustrations in the book. Brett patiently and effectively rendered my unusual specifications on good and bad posture.

Tom Tworek, for shooting and editing all of the instructional photographs. His good humor and reassuring manner made the photo-shoots a pleasure.

Prudence Breitrose, for helping re-edit the entire book and much improving it.

Cara Rosaen, for challenging me to refine my arguments in the Foundations chapter and then helping search the medical literature to enable me to do so.

Dan Leemon, for the name "Remember When It Didn't Hurt."

Deborah Addicott, for being the model for Lesson 6.

Janetti Marotta, for being my writing buddy during the year in which I wrote the first draft of the book.

Grant Barnes, Gertrude Bock, William Carter, Bridget Conrad, Laila Craveiro, Benjamin Davidson, Sheila dela Rosa, Julie Dorsey, DeWitt Durham, Elaine Gradman, Kevin Johnson, Leah McGarrigle, Susan Mellen, Michele Raffin, David Riggs, Beth Siegelman, Camille Spar, Julie Stanford, and Anne White, for valuable feedback on the content of the book.

Margo Davis, Angela Fischer/photokunst, Donald Greig, Ian Mackenzie, Randy Mont-Reynaud, Sandra Starkey-Simon, the family of Gerard Mackworth-Young, Dreamstime, iStockphoto, Shutterstock, and the Library of Congress for images that appear in the book.

Susan Adams, Deborah Addicott, Teresa Arnold, Suruchi Bhutani, Brian Danitz, Tushar Dave, Sheila dela Rosa, Vinod Dham, DeWitt Durham, Trish Hayes-Danitz, Miri Hutcherson, Kevin Johnson, Chloe Kamprath, Dan Leemon, Alon Maor, Michele Raffin, T.M. Ravi, Evan Roberts, Cara Rosaen, Beth Siegelman, Julie Stanford, and Susan Wojcicki, for valuable advice on business matters related to the book.

The hundreds of subjects who let me photograph them, talk to them, and use their pictures for my work.

Brian, Maya, Nathan, and Monisha White. No author has had a more supportive family.

CONTENTS

FOREWORD xv
PREFACE xvii

FOUNDATIONS 2
BACK PAIN   6
WHAT WE BLAME   6
   STANDING UPRIGHT?   6
   SEDENTARY LIVES?   7
   STRESS?   8
   WEIGHT AND HEIGHT?   9
   AGE?   10
THE REAL CAUSE   10
   LOSS OF KINESTHETIC TRADITION   13
   INFLUENCE OF THE FASHION INDUSTRY   15
THE EFFECT ON OUR BACKS   16
MOVING OUT OF MISERY   17
HOW IT WORKS   17
WHAT DOES GOOD POSTURE LOOK LIKE?   18
   ANTEVERTED PELVIS   20
   A GENTLY CURVED, ELONGATED SPINE   21
   EVERY BONE IN ITS NATURAL PLACE   22
   USING MUSCLES MORE THAN JOINTS   23
   MUSCLES FULLY RELAXED WHEN NOT WORKING   23
   BREATHING AS A THERAPEUTIC EXERCISE   23
IT WORKS!   24

ORIENTATION 26
FOLLOW THE LESSON SEQUENCE   28
   HERNIATED DISC   28
   HIGH IMPACT ACTIVITIES   28
   BENDING ACTIVITIES   28
ALLOW TIME TO CHANGE   28
KNOW WHAT TO EXPECT   29
   HOW QUICKLY CAN I EXPECT RESULTS?   29
   HOW LONG SHOULD EACH LESSON TAKE?   29
   HOW DIFFICULT ARE THE LESSONS?   29
UNDERSTAND HOW THE LESSONS ARE ORGANIZED   29
RECOGNIZE YOUR PROGRESS   30
BARRIERS TO SUCCESS   30

LESSON 1: STRETCHSITTING 32
BENEFITS   36
INSTRUCTIONS   38
INDICATIONS OF IMPROVEMENT   48

TROUBLESHOOTING   48
    FEELING OVERLY STRETCHED   48
    UNABLE TO STRETCH THE SPINE   48
    DISCOMFORT AT POINT OF CONTACT   49
    INADEQUATE CHAIR   49
FURTHER INFORMATION   49
    SHOULDER REPOSITIONING   49
    COMMENTS ON LUMBAR CUSHIONS   50
SITTING IN A CAR   50
    FASHIONING A BACKREST   51
    CHECKING YOUR POSITION   51
RECAP   53

LESSON 2: STRETCHLYING ON YOUR BACK 54
BENEFITS   57
INSTRUCTIONS   58
INDICATIONS OF IMPROVEMENT   64
TROUBLESHOOTING   64
    FEELING PAIN OR DISCOMFORT IN THE LOW BACK   64
    FEELING PAIN OR DISCOMFORT IN THE NECK   64
    FEELING DISCOMFORT AT A POINT OF CONTACT WITH THE BED   65
    SNORING   65
    FEELINGS OF EXPOSURE   65
FURTHER INFORMATION   65
    BEDS   65
    PILLOWS   65
    CERVICAL PILLOWS / ROLLS   66
RECAP   67

LESSON 3: STACKSITTING 68
THE WEDGE   71
THE ANTEVERTED PELVIS   72
BENEFITS   73
INSTRUCTIONS   74
INDICATIONS OF IMPROVEMENT   88
TROUBLESHOOTING   88
    PAIN IN THE LOW BACK   88
    SORENESS IN THE LOW BACK   88
    WEDGE NOT AVAILABLE   88
    INELEGANT MOVEMENT   88
    CHANGED LINE OF VISION   89
FURTHER INFORMATION   89
    CONFLICTING GUIDELINES   89
    DISTINCTION BETWEEN TIPPING THE PELVIS AND SWAYING THE BACK   89
    CHAIRS   90
    FLOOR   91
RECAP   93

LESSON 4: STRETCHLYING ON YOUR SIDE 94
BENEFITS   97
INSTRUCTIONS   98

INDICATIONS OF IMPROVEMENT   106
TROUBLESHOOTING   106
    YOU CAN'T FALL ASLEEP   106
    YOUR BODY DOESN'T HOLD THE POSITION THROUGH THE NIGHT   106
    YOU ARE UNCOMFORTABLE IN THIS POSITION   106
FURTHER INFORMATION   107
    SLEEPING ON YOUR STOMACH   107
    WHAT TO DO WITH YOUR LEGS   108
RECAP   109

LESSON 5: USING YOUR INNER CORSET   110
BENEFITS   114
INSTRUCTIONS   116
INDICATIONS OF IMPROVEMENT   122
TROUBLESHOOTING   122
    SWAYING THE LOW BACK   122
    DIFFICULTY BREATHING   122
FURTHER INFORMATION   122
    LENGTHENING BY CONTRACTING   122
    JUMPING   123
    REACHING ABOVE YOUR HEAD   123
    PROTECTING YOUR NECK   124
    USING AN EXTERNAL CORSET   124
RECAP   127

LESSON 6: TALLSTANDING   128
BENEFITS   131
INSTRUCTIONS   134
INDICATIONS OF IMPROVEMENT   142
TROUBLESHOOTING   142
    UNABLE TO CONTRACT THE FOOT ARCH   142
    DIFFICULTY SHIFTING WEIGHT ONTO HEELS   142
    PROBLEMS ALIGNING THE SHOULDERS   143
    INABILITY TO SENSE YOUR VERTICAL AXIS   143
FURTHER INFORMATION   144
    ARM POSITION   144
    WEIGHT ON THE HEELS   145
    NATURAL ARCHES OF THE FEET   145
    BARE FEET   146
    PREGNANCY   146
    INSOLES   146
    SHOES   146
    SPINE CONTOUR CONFUSION   146
RECAP   149

LESSON 7: HIP-HINGING   150
ANATOMY OF A BACKACHE...   153
... AND HOW TO AVOID IT   153

BENEFITS 155

COMPARING DIFFERENT BENDING STYLES 155

INSTRUCTIONS 156

INDICATIONS OF IMPROVEMENT 162

TROUBLESHOOTING 162

    BENDING IS PAINFUL 162

    THE GROOVE IN YOUR LOW BACK DISAPPEARS AS YOU BEND 162

    THE GROOVE IN YOUR LOW BACK GETS DEEPER AS YOU BEND 163

FURTHER INFORMATION 163

    HAMSTRING FLEXIBILITY 163

    BENDING FOR EXTENDED PERIODS 164

    BENDING WHILE SITTING 164

    EXTRA WEIGHT 164

    HIP-HINGING FOR ATHLETIC ADVANTAGE 164

    TRAINING CHILDREN TO HIP-HINGE 165

RECAP 167

LESSON 8: GLIDEWALKING 168

BENEFITS 172

INSTRUCTIONS 174

INDICATIONS OF IMPROVEMENT 190

TROUBLESHOOTING 190

    FEELING THAT YOU ARE LEANING FORWARD 190

    TENDENCY TO TUCK OR LEAD WIITH THE PELVIS 190

    UNABLE TO COORDINATE BUTTOCK CONTRACTION AND FORWARD THRUST 190

    DIFFICULTY LEAVING BACK HEEL ON THE FLOOR 190

    LOSING TRACK OF YOUR POSTURE 190

    CANNOT COORDINATE ALL THE ELEMENTS OF GLIDEWALKING 191

FURTHER INFORMATION 191

    WALKING ON ONE LINE 191

    GETTING EXTRA POWER IN YOUR STRIDE 192

    RUNNING LIKE A KENYAN 192

RECAP 193

APPENDIX 1: OPTIONAL EXERCISES 195

STRENGTHENING THE TORSO MUSCLES 197

    STRENGTHENING THE ABDOMINAL MUSCLES 197

    STRENGTHENING THE DEEP MUSCLES OF THE BACK 204

STRENGTHENING AND STRETCHING THE MUSCLES IN THE SHOULDER AREA 205

STRENGTHENING THE NECK MUSCLES 207

STRETCHING THE NECK MUSCLES 207

STRETCHING THE KEY MUSCLES THAT CONNECT THE TORSO AND LEGS 208

    STRETCHING THE HAMSTRINGS 208

    STRETCHING THE EXTERNAL HIP ROTATOR MUSCLES 210

    LENGTHENING THE PSOAS 210

STRENGTHENING KEY MUSCLES USED IN WALKING 211

    STRENGTHENING THE ARCH MUSCLES 211

STRENGTHENING THE GLUTEUS MEDIUS MUSCLES   213
STRENGTHENING THE TIBIALIS ANTERIOR   214

TROUBLESHOOTING   215
  STIFFNESS OR PAIN   215
  LACK OF IMPROVEMENT   215
  FAILURE TO EXERCISE   215
FURTHER INFORMATION   215

APPENDIX 2: ANATOMY 217

GLOSSARY 220

BIBLIOGRAPHY 223

INDEX 224

SUMMARY GUIDE 226

FOREWORD

On a crisp, clear day in January, I invited my husband and daughter to take a hike up Windy Hill, one of the steepest trails in the Bay Area. It was a challenge, since I hadn't attempted the hike for over a year. But when my husband and daughter stopped half way up, I was the one who kept going, motoring up that trail with no difficulty, in spite of my bulky bag. When I returned to my family waiting below, I realized what a gift Esther Gokhale had given me! Her techniques had enabled me to complete the hike with much less effort than it would have taken the year before.

As a doctor in Internal Medicine, I have seen many patients with chronic back and neck problems in my 24 years of practice, and I have always been on the lookout for new methods of treatment. In December 2005, I found one. Esther Gokhale had been invited to tell my department at the Palo Alto Medical Clinic about her approach to the prevention and treatment of spinal problems. When I walked into the conference room, I thought at first that this erudite, soft-spoken young woman was giving an Art History seminar instead of a dry medical lecture: projected on the screen were beautiful torsos from antiquity and exquisite photographs from around the world, giving examples of human posture from prehistoric times to the present.

I was riveted. As Esther demonstrated, our anatomical stance had been preserved for thousands of years, only to change radically in the past century. Possible reasons for this shift are fascinating, but ultimately irrelevant. The consequences, however, are significant, providing a clue to some of our society's most common ailments: the back and neck pains that we suffer far more than our ancestors or our counterparts in less industrialized societies.

This was a big "ah-ha" moment for me, and I wanted to learn more. With a colleague, I enrolled in Esther's posture class, and in six one-hour sessions, I learned her simple steps for restoring the spine to its natural alignment. I was astonished by how easily these steps could be integrated into my busy life. I could lengthen my spine as I slept, drove to work, walked to my office, sat at my desk, worked on the computer, and sat on a stool talking to my patients. Within weeks, I was sleeping better, I had more energy, and my neck no longer ached. I also had a new sense of well-being. My patients and colleagues commented on how well I looked and asked me if I had lost weight – all this while I was entering menopause!

I referred my 85 year-old mother-in-law, who has a withered left side from childhood polio, severe osteoporosis, and arthritis. Could Esther's program help someone who could only move bent over a walker? Within one session, I had my answer. My mother-in-law was already sitting straighter, and by the end of the program, for the first time in years, she had learned to pick herself up from the floor unassisted, in case of a fall. I realized that Esther was really onto something, and that it is never too late to reverse the effects of decades of "poor" posture. Imagine what could be achieved if this knowledge were more widely disseminated – if teenagers could establish healthy body postures that would support them throughout their lives!

I began referring patients to Esther, as did many of my colleagues. Some of the results were astonishing, especially in patients whose problems had seemed intractable. For example, one woman in her 80s was so severely arthritic that for years she had been unable to write. After a few sessions with Esther, she was writing again.

My colleagues and I urged Esther to make her techniques available to a wider audience through this book. The techniques are simple to learn and superbly suited to a world that prizes the quick fix, since they require no special equipment, membership fees, coaches, or athletic ability. Even a bent-over, arthritic 85-year-old can follow the step-by-step instructions.

How does Esther's method work? Basically, by restoring the spine to its optimal length, and the rest of the body's architecture to its optimal position. For the elderly, this helps counteract the consequences of aging and gravity on the spine, such as shorter stature, smaller lung capacity, decreased abdominal cavity (and the concomitant problems of sluggish bowels and constipation, urinary frequency and urge-incontinence). For people of all ages, the method improves balance, pulmonary function, circulation to the limbs, and spinal architecture. It facilitates body awareness and a sense of empowerment because the steps are so easy to perform and because the results accrue from day one.

Since participating in Esther's program I look at the human skeleton in a whole new way. I have come to see how its elegant design dictates the function of our structural underpinnings, and can affect the efficiency of every part of us. For example, despite wearing sensible shoes, I have had bunions all my adult life. After working with Esther, I realized I was walking with the majority of my weight on my forefoot instead of on the far denser and sturdier heel bone. Since I have learned the "glidewalking" technique that you will find in this book, the heavier part of my skeleton absorbs more of the weight. Similarly, being in the "tail out" position when I sit is far more comfortable, helping me keep my back straight and my neck long. I value being able to work on my "inner corset" through activities of daily living, rather than by sweating and straining in a gym.

As one of my colleagues declared, I have become a true believer. I am convinced that the dramatic postural changes that have occurred in our society over the last hundred years can be reversed, and that we can return to a healthy, natural style with the help of Esther's insights and techniques. If enough of us take advantage of her program and follow the simple steps in this book, we will see a new generation of people with beautiful posture and strong supple bodies, able to work and play without pain long into old age.

Deirdre Stegman, M.D.,
Palo Alto Medical Foundation, CA

PREFACE

For some, a pain-free life is only a memory, but it doesn't have to be. Through my experience in healing my own back pain, coupled with extensive training and research, I have developed a technique to alleviate back pain—the Gokhale Method^{SM}. It has been a privilege and a pleasure to help thousands of people re-learn the way their bodies were designed to move—gracefully and with ease. I have spent fifteen years teaching the technique, honing it for clarity and efficiency, and am delighted to present it here for general use.

My own back pain started in college while doing a yoga pose. I almost immediately experienced back spasms, which fortunately resolved with bed rest and muscle relaxants. A few years later I injured my back again. This time, I needed five days of bed rest to recover. I began a regimen of weight training to help my back and soon returned to a physically active life.

Then, when I was nine months pregnant with my first child, the pain returned with an insidious onset of sciatica. I was told the pain would dissipate after the baby was born. It did not; in fact, it grew worse. Eventually I could not lie down for more than two hours at a time. I spent the midnight hours walking my neighborhood to alleviate the pain. When my baby was a year old, I underwent back surgery (specifically an L5-S1 laminectomy/discectomy) for a badly herniated disc. For several months post-surgery, I had a relatively pain-free life, although I could not lift or carry my daughter, and was advised to have no more children. I had already decided that, rather than risk months of hellish pain again, my first child would be my last. Within 12 months of my surgery, the pain returned and my doctors recommended further surgery. Instead, I decided to find my own path out of misery and to begin my own deeper research into the causes and treatments for back pain.

I learned about L'Institut d'Aplomb in Paris, France, where Noelle Perez teaches an anthropologically-based posture modification technique. Her theory is that we in industrialized countries don't use our bodies well, that this misuse can cause pain and damage, and that we have much to learn from people in traditional cultures. The theory resonated with my childhood memories from growing up in India. I remembered listening to my Dutch mother marvel at how gracefully our Indian maid went about her duties and how easily the laborers in the street carried their burdens. Classes in

Noelle's technique diminished my back pain significantly, and I spent five years training to become certified in Aplomb®. Spurred on by what I learned, I attended courses at Stanford University Medical School and Department of Anthropology. I visited countries in Europe, Asia, Africa, and South America observing, photographing, filming, and interviewing people without back pain. I incorporated teachings from other disciplines, added elements from my field research, and created a unique, systematic method for helping people efficiently transform their posture and return to physically active lives. I offered my method to my acupuncture patients who suffered from musculo-skeletal problems. The results were stunning, and I began to share my method with a larger audience.

Many physicians now refer their back patients to me, and almost all the patients start to improve from the first lesson. In many cases the results are dramatic (see page 24).

But then there are the people who can't come to see me, people who call me from the East Coast or the Midwest, perhaps friends or relatives of my patients, who are suffering terribly and need help. For years, I have wished there were a book that I could send them with step-by-step instructions and demonstrations of my technique.

And here it is.

Esther Gokhale,
Stanford, CA, 2007

FOUNDATIONS

Your body's way back to pain-free living

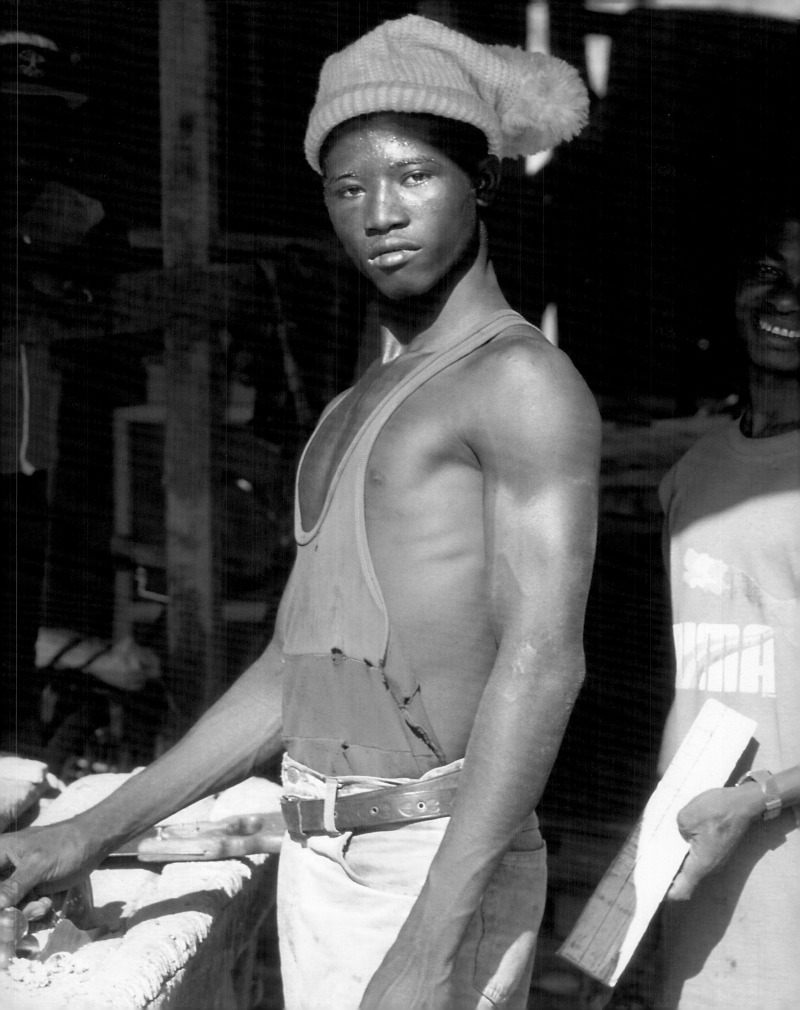

We are marvelously designed creatures. We have inherent grace and strength, like every other creature on the planet. We have evolved to sit, walk, run, jump, climb, carry, and even dance without pain. If we respect our natural design, our bodies heal spontaneously, and we can function well for close to a century. Indeed, there are many populations where most people live painlessly into old age (fig.F-1).[1-9]

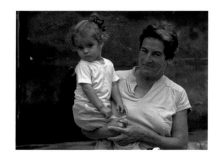

This grandmother carries her grandchild with ease (Brazil).

fig.F-1

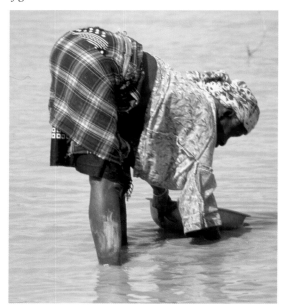

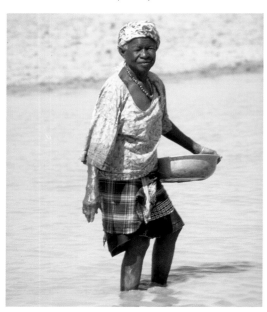

This older woman bends to gather water chestnuts for seven to nine hours a day, but reports no pain (Burkina Faso).

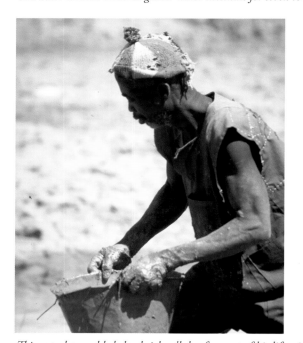

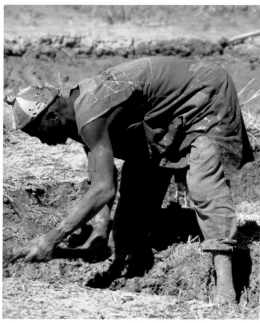

This man has molded clay bricks all day for most of his life with no negative physical impact (Burkina Faso).

Why, then, do so many people in our culture suffer back pain and other musculo-skeletal ills? The problem is that we arrive on the planet without a user's manual. We depend on our culture to teach and support us. And the culture in industrialized societies has not been teaching or supporting us very well (fig.F-2). If we have pain and musculo-skeletal problems, we need to look first at the laws of nature we are disrespecting, the blueprint for our skeletal structure we are disregarding, the pieces of our genetic code we are ignoring. This book introduces you to a technique that teaches and supports you in a way that our culture no longer does, so that you can live a normal, pain-free life.

fig.F-2

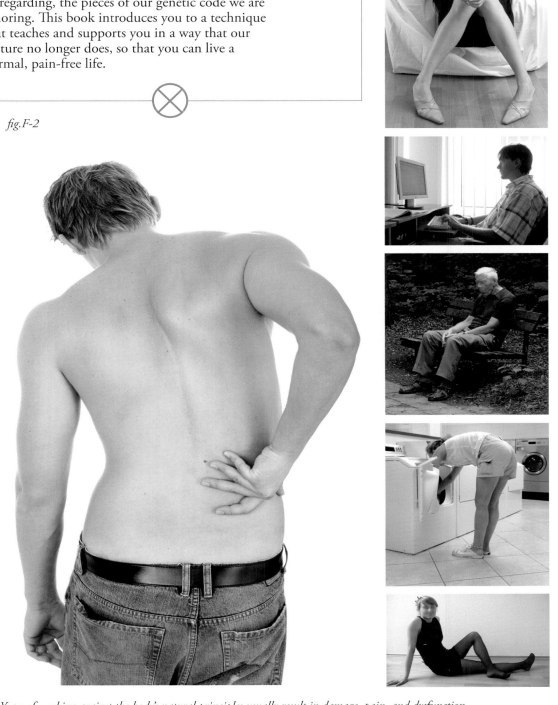

Years of working against the body's natural principles usually result in damage, pain, and dysfunction.

BACK PAIN

If you suffer back pain, you are not alone. In industrialized societies, back pain has reached epidemic proportions. Consider these statistics for the United States:

• Approximately 80 percent of individuals in the general population will have at least one episode of low back pain during their lifetime [10,11].

• Back pain lasting at least two weeks affects approximately one in seven adults each year. [11]

• Back pain is the second leading symptom for physician visits in the United States. [12]

• By age 15, more than 60% of all adolescents have experienced back and/or neck pain. [13]

• Back pain is the leading cause of work-related disability, accounting for 33 percent of all workers' compensation costs. [11]

• Total direct and indirect costs for treatment of low back pain are estimated to be $100 billion annually. [14]

Every year tens of thousands of patients undergo major back surgery without any benefit. By using Esther Gokhale's novel techniques, many of these patients can avoid such needless and expensive medical procedures, and quickly return to a pain-free life.

John Adler, M.D., Neurosurgeon, Stanford University Medical Clinic, Stanford, CA

After back surgery in 1991, I was still in excruciating pain and lived with prescription pain medication on a daily basis. Esther Gokhale changed all that. I no longer have any neck pain or back pain and I no longer use any pain medication.

Stacia Hurley, Project Manager, Concentric Network, CA

The Gokhale Method[SM] helped me eradicate my lower back pain, even though surgery was recommended. It helped me understand the origins of my pain and taught me proper posture techniques (walking, sitting, sleeping) to achieve long-term healing and well-being of body and mind.

Elfi Altendorfer, Redwood City, CA

WHAT WE BLAME

Among the most commonly cited causes for our high rates of back pain are that we are not designed to stand upright, we are too sedentary, we endure too much stress, we've grown too tall or too heavy for our backs, and we wear out with age. But are these factors really the problem?

STANDING UPRIGHT?

The argument goes that our spines have not evolved sufficiently to carry the weight of our upper bodies, necks, and heads without strain or damage. [15] By this reasoning, we should all be suffering back pain. Yet there are whole populations where the incidence is very low. [1-9]

Five and a half million years of being upright is plenty of time—even by evolutionary standards—for our spines to adapt and accommodate the "new" burden of our upper bodies. I believe that the problem is not an evolutionary flaw, but a cultural one. The cause of our pain is not *that* we stand upright, but *how* we stand upright (figs.F-3, F-4).

People have been telling me to stand up straight all my life. It never made any sense until Esther showed me how.

Jessica Ruvinsky, writer, New York, NY

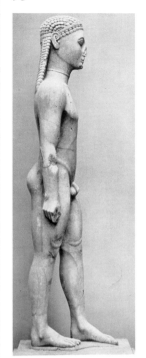
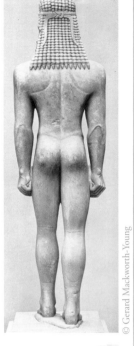

fig.F-3

© Gerard Mackworth-Young

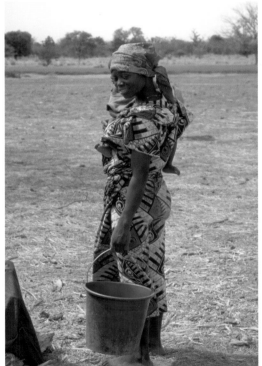

People from diverse cultures exhibit healthy upright posture (Greece, Burkina Faso).

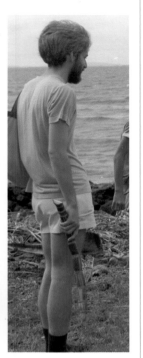

fig.F-4

Our problem is not that we stand upright, but how we stand upright.

SEDENTARY LIVES?

Another frequently cited excuse for our back pain is our sedentary way of life: unlike people in many parts of the world, most workers in industrialized societies earn their living sitting down. Yet statistics show that in industrialized societies manual laborers have an even higher incidence of low back pain than sedentary workers.[16] This suggests that switching from sedentary jobs to more physical ones would not solve our back problems.

In my travels in Burkina Faso, Ecuador, and India, I encountered numerous sedentary workers including potters, basket makers, and weavers, who spend long hours sitting and yet do not suffer from nearly as many back problems as we do (fig.F-5). In our culture as well, some people manage long hours in front of computer screens without negative consequences to their backs. In fact, recent medical statistics call into question the agreed-upon philosophy that static sitting at work is a risk factor for low back pain.[17] Again, I believe that it isn't *that* we sit but *how* we sit that causes our problems (fig.F-6).

My students, after they have learned a few simple relevant techniques, usually find sitting extremely comfortable, even if it previously caused them pain.

I found Esther's method of "stacksitting" amazingly comfortable, even for long periods. Before, so-called "good posture" had always felt unnatural, as well as a tremendous amount of work. Now, I tend to be uncomfortable in a slumped position, and instinctively search for the most lengthened, relaxed position in whatever I'm doing.

Barbara Kerckhoff,
Palo Alto, CA

fig.F-6

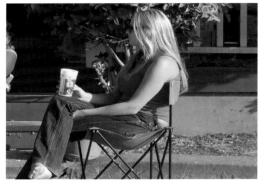

Hunched sitting (USA)

fig.F-5

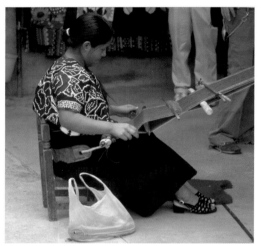

Weaving cloth (Mexico)

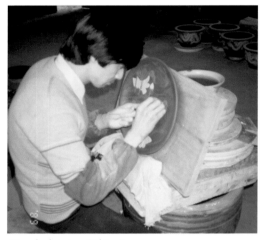

Hunched sitting (China)
It isn't that we sit, but how we sit that causes our problems.

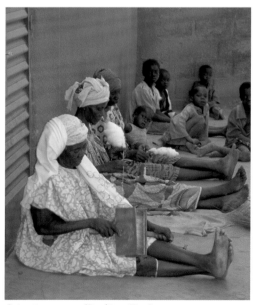

Spinning cotton (Burkina Faso)
These sedentary workers have healthy posture and report no back pain.

STRESS?

While stress is a risk factor for back pain,[15] it is possible to address physical pain independently from stress. Stress correlates with pain, but doesn't have to cause it. If you have stress-related back pain, you can lessen your pain by learning physical relaxation even if you are not able to resolve your stress. In fact, learning positions that are physically relaxing can help you deal better with mental and emotional stress.

I used to have a lot of tension in my neck and shoulders. Since doing the posture work, I can't remember the last time I've had any discomfort at all.

Kathy Uros, VP, Charles Schwab & Co.,
San Francisco, CA

WEIGHT AND HEIGHT?

Extra weight challenges the entire skeleton and enormous extra weight is certainly unhealthy. A moderate amount of excess weight, however, need not cause serious musculo-skeletal problems (fig.F-7).[18] It is when an individual lacks good alignment that even a small amount of extra weight can be disproportionately damaging because it torques the spine.

A building that is built true is not unstable, even if it is bulky; but if it is even slightly skewed, the extra bulk exerts great strains on the underlying structure. Similarly, if the spine is properly aligned, it will tolerate moderate amounts of extra weight without damage; if the spine is poorly aligned, every degree of misalignment causes a large increase in stress. For people who carry extra weight and experience back pain, learning proper alignment may provide a faster and more direct solution to their back pain than losing the extra weight.

Just as excess weight can challenge the skeletal system, so can unusual height. Similar logic applies: on a poorly aligned skeleton, extra height significantly stresses the spine; on a well-aligned skeleton, extra height need not cause damage.[19] Consider the Masai, who are usually well over six feet tall, but are spared our epidemic of back pain.[20]

Episodes of incapacitating pain became more frequent as the years went by, even though I pretty conscientiously followed recommendations of doctors and physical therapists who prescribed the usual exercise regimes. When the pain became unbearable I spent from one to ten days flat on my back in bed, taking pain medications, a muscle relaxant, and cursing my feeble and somewhat overweight body.

Since taking the posture class over ten years ago, I have had no recurrence of severe back pain, and have been able to immediately relieve small pains by one of Esther's simple techniques. No more pain pills, no more muscle relaxants.

Grant Barnes, Director Emeritus, Stanford University Press, Sebastopol, CA

I am over 6'3" and had the common problem of tall people in tending to slouch. Back pain was an everyday fact of life, and influenced what I could and could not do. Since working with the Gokhale Method℠, I no longer slouch and back pain no longer restricts me from any activity.

Charles Bacon, Senior Research Geologist, USGS, Menlo Park, CA

fig.F-7

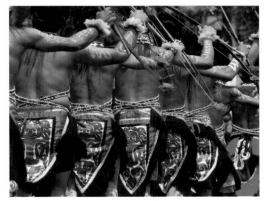

(Papua New Guinea)

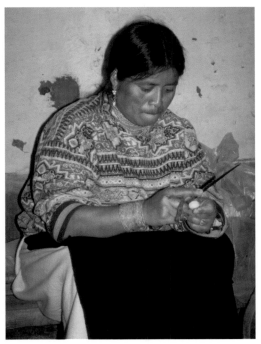

(Ecuador)

Extra weight does not condemn people to back pain. In many cultures, full-bodied people carry their extra weight without great difficulty.

AGE?

Many people think that age is the biggest contributor to back pain. Certainly with age our bones and muscles weaken; however, the same is true for all humanity. If we use our bodies wisely, normal wear and tear should not incapacitate us. The Burkina brickmaker in figure F-8a shows what is possible even in advanced age. He spends numerous hours every day digging clay, mixing it with straw, and fashioning it into bricks using a wood mold. In some low-income, rural communities, 80-90% of workers are laborers who often carry heavy weights on their backs and heads and may work well into old age. Yet their rates of low back pain are 50-75% less than in higher-income, industrialized populations.[1]

> I am 85 years old and in the last couple of years have had low back pain when doing kitchen work and other chores. I assumed this was because of my age. I was pleasantly surprised to learn from the Gokhale Method [SM] that this kind of back pain is not inevitable. I now do my household chores without any pain at all. I also got rid of my knee pain and walk faster.
>
> Gertrude Bock,
> Palo Alto, CA

> Esther Gokhale's method makes a lifetime of postural habits easy to transform, and fun, too. At 60, I thought it was too late. Through this approach, both joyful and scientific, my body now appears from the outside as it feels from the inside, strong and whole.
>
> Joan Ruvinsky,
> Yoga teacher
> Montreal, Canada

fig. F-8

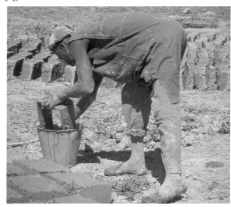

a. This brickmaker works long hours making bricks from straw and clay despite his age (Burkina Faso).

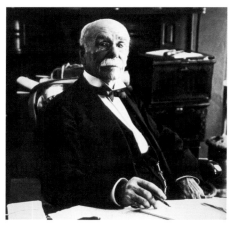

b. The clerk in this photograph from the turn of the century is not young but works from "sun up to sun down six days a week" (USA).

THE REAL CAUSE

Scientific research substantiates the following risk factors for back pain: genetics,[21, 22] psychosocial stress, exposure to vibration, inadequate physical fitness, strenuous body positioning (bending, twisting, static standing), age,[15] height (only in the case of sciatica),[19] smoking,[23] and other health conditions (such as arthritis, infections, tumors, and osteoporosis).[25] I believe that the biggest risk factor for back pain, as yet unidentified and underappreciated, is posture.

Many of these known risk factors can be mitigated by good posture. People with good posture can better withstand the effects of whole-body vibration, strenuous body positioning, weight, height, age, and even genetic predisposition to disc degeneration. Without good posture, however, some of the above factors, especially genetics, become very significant.

Much of our back pain results from how we hold ourselves and how we move. We have lost sight of what constitutes healthy posture; in fact, many popular guidelines for "good posture" do more harm than good. To find a model for healthy posture, we need to return to the ways of moving that were normal for us in earlier times and that are still normal for people in many cultures.

Until the 20th century, debilitating back pain was not common in our society. Today, back pain is more than twice as common as it was in 1950.[25] Shortly after World War I, a confluence of trends began a vicious cycle that continues today. Compare the pictures of individuals taken at the end of the 19th century (fig.F-9) with that from the mid-20th century (fig.F-10). The change is dramatic. Notice that, compared with the people in the earlier images, after the 1920's, people began to thrust their pelvises and necks forward, and hunch or round their shoulders. It became fashionable to slouch.

Even more startling is a comparison of spine illustrations from two medical textbooks, one published in 1911 (fig. F-11a), the other in 1990 (fig.F-11b). Whereas the 1911 illustration shows gently curved, elongated low back (lumbar) and upper back (thoracic) spinal contours, the later drawing shows significantly increased curvature both in the lumbar and thoracic spine. The shape of the spine in the 1911 illustration is shared not only by our ancestors, but also by adults in traditional cultures today (fig.F-3), and young children the world over (fig.F-12). The consistency across generations, cultures, geography, and age provides compelling evidence that this is indeed the natural shape of the human spine. Here is a dramatic clue to the cause of our current back pain epidemic. Clearly, a mere 80 years of human history is not sufficient to account for any substantial genetic alteration of something as basic as the shape of our spines. What we are seeing is a cultural drift away from our natural design and an ancient and widespread kinesthetic tradition – the tradition of movement and posture handed down through earlier generations.

So, what is the cause of this cultural drift? This is a matter for research, but I conjecture that two forces play an important role: a disruption in the link between generations in our culture, and the influence of the fashion industry.

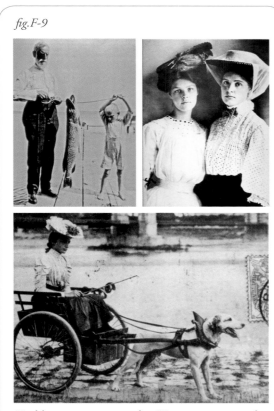

fig.F-9

Healthy posture was typical in Western societies until the late 19th and early 20th centuries (USA).

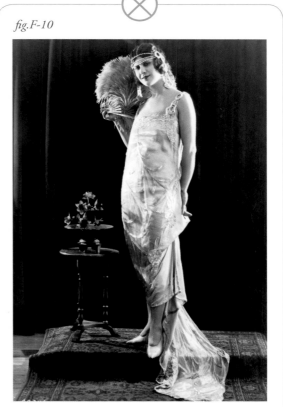

fig.F-10

Beginning in the 1920's, it became fashionable to slouch

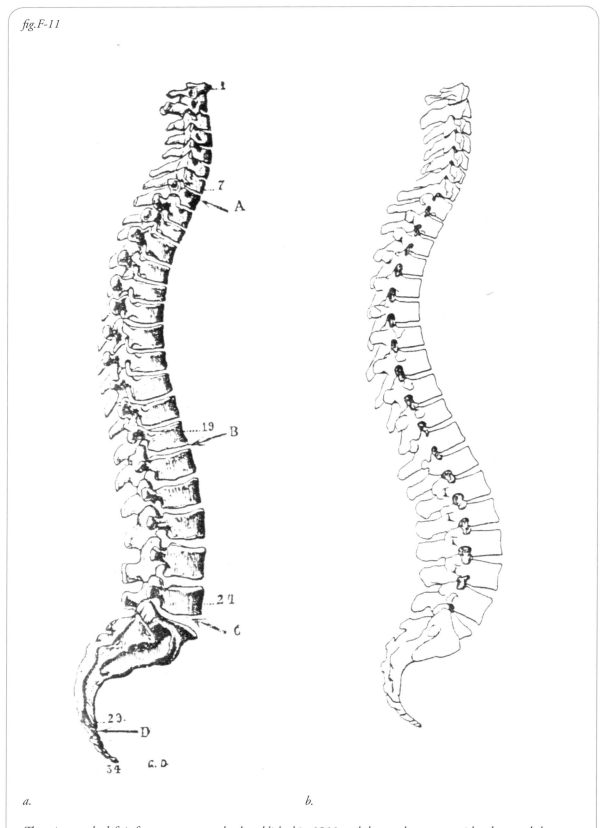

fig.F-11

a.

b.

The spine on the left is from an anatomy book published in 1911 and shows what was considered normal then. The spine on the right is copied from an anatomy book published in 1990 and shows what is considered normal spinal curvature today. Notice the marked shift in the degree of curvature throughout the spine and especially in the low back (lumbar) area.

fig.F-12

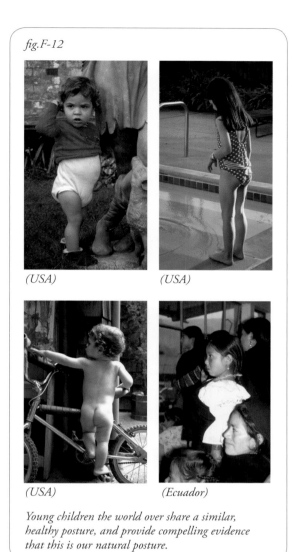

(USA)   *(USA)*

(USA)   *(Ecuador)*

Young children the world over share a similar, healthy posture, and provide compelling evidence that this is our natural posture.

fig.F-13

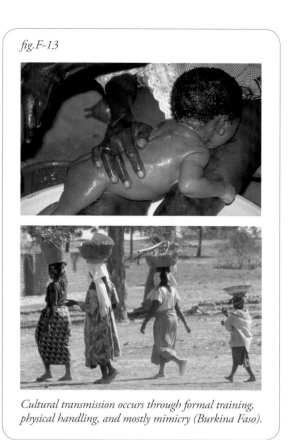

Cultural transmission occurs through formal training, physical handling, and mostly mimicry (Burkina Faso).

LOSS OF KINESTHETIC TRADITION

In modern industrial societies, many families have become geographically dispersed, with couples raising their children far away from parents and grandparents. This has led to a break in cultural support and the handing down of kinesthetic tradition. By contrast, in tribal Africa, rural Portugal, village India, and other traditional societies, families are not dispersed and kinesthetic traditions remain intact. Though human beings share a fine blueprint for physical well-being, it takes cultural support, especially in the formative years, to pass body wisdom from one generation to the next. Cultural support comes in the form of grandparents showing parents how to carry their children, of teachers guiding their students to sit well in class, of children mimicking parents as they bend to gather food (fig.F-13).

Whereas certain cultural knowledge is easily transmitted by modern means of communication, kinesthetic knowledge needs physical proximity and repeated visual cueing. When the kinesthetic line is broken, we improvise each action rather than draw on the wisdom of thousands of generations.

Especially important among our kinesthetic traditions are those relating to children, since it is during the crucial early years that posture and movement patterns are etched into the brain. These traditions include how to hold a child while nursing, how to carry a child, and how to teach a child to sit well (fig.F-14). Today's parents and grandparents have lost the generational wisdom for performing these actions well (fig.F-15) and today's children are the worse for it (fig.F-16).

Often, the only posture guideline children receive today is an occasional admonition to "sit up straight." Not knowing how to sit well, most children briefly adopt a stiff pose with tension in the low back, but quickly tire of it and revert to slouching. Our popular wisdom no longer includes good postural knowledge.

Even our medical experts are not well-informed about the elements of good posture and how to implement them. The medical establishment has lost sight of what truly ideal posture is, and mistakes the current average as normal or even ideal. Medical recommendations, interventions, and devices such as lumbar support cushions (page 50), cervical pillows (page 66), and TLSO body casts (page 125) reflect and perpetuate this cultural drift. They tend to accentuate excessive curvature in the small of the back (upper lumbar spine) and the neck (cervical spine), and flatten the natural *lumbo-sacral curve.*

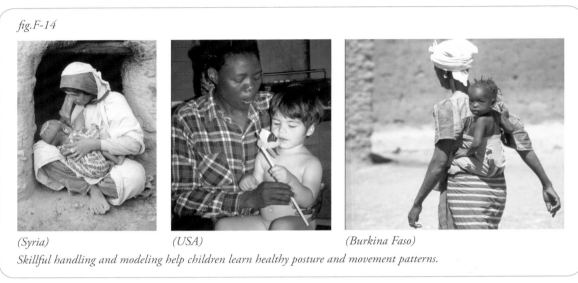

fig.F-14

(Syria)   (USA)   (Burkina Faso)

Skillful handling and modeling help children learn healthy posture and movement patterns.

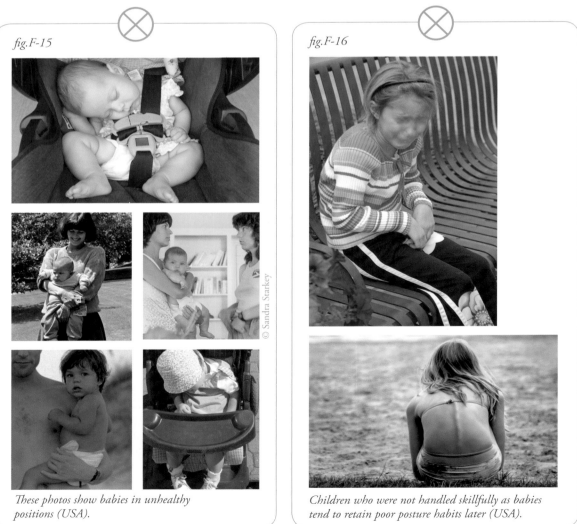

fig.F-15

© Sandra Starkey

These photos show babies in unhealthy positions (USA).

fig.F-16

Children who were not handled skillfully as babies tend to retain poor posture habits later (USA).

I urge you to take a class from her, or hear her presentation, so that your world can be opened like mine was, to a better understanding of back health and overall physical well being. I am constantly teaching Esther's vision (as best I can) to my patients. I agree with her that our traditional teaching of how to care for backs is not optimal. I think her vision is better. I think it is right.

Jessica Davidson, M.D., Internal Medicine, Palo Alto Medical Foundation, Palo Alto, CA

I came from Sweden to visit my mother in Palo Alto and was surprised to see that she was standing and sitting straighter and generally feeling better. This piqued my interest in the Gokhale Method ℠*, since I am a naturopathic physician and can always use new ways to help my patients.*

Letting my behind stick out, instead of keeping it tucked as I was taught before, was the hardest to remember. The surprising thing was that the new posture became natural very quickly. After a few days, I realized that the tension in my neck had disappeared. Slumping and tucking my behind became uncomfortable.

I realized why I had been having so many aches and pains doing massage all day. When the posture is right it feels relaxed. That amazes me.

Catherine Bock-Nilsson, Naturopathic Physician, Sweden

INFLUENCE OF THE FASHION INDUSTRY

Another major contributor to our posture drift is the fashion industry. Around World War I, fashions in clothing and furniture converged to transform the conception of the human figure. In a matter of a few years, French fashion magazines moved from showing models with natural posture (fig.F-17) to showing ones with severely distorted frames, tucked pelvises, slouched shoulders, and protruding necks (fig.F-18) – much like the runway models of today. The fashion industry in the 1920's promoted this posture as relaxed, casual, and new, as opposed to classical posture, which was reframed as stiff, rigid, and passé. Furniture styles also shifted in the 1920's (figs.F-19, F-20) reinforcing the trend towards slouching in the name of comfort and ease. The Mies van der Rohe chair is an early example of furniture that tucks the pelvis and strongly distorts the spine. Many modern chairs do the same (fig.3-15, on page 90).

fig.F-17

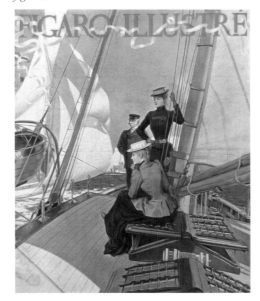

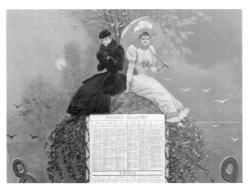

French fashion magazines from before World War I depict healthy posture.

fig.F-18

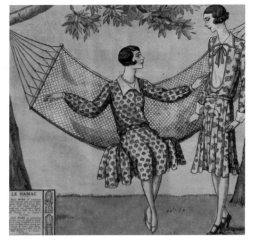

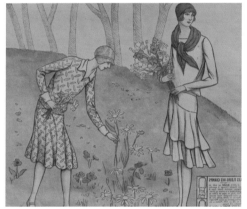

French fashion magazines from the 1920's and later show slouching as chic.

fig.F-19

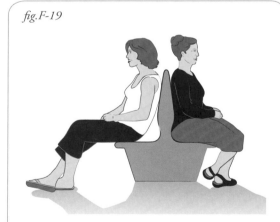

This sketch of passengers on a Portuguese barge shows a seat constructed when the average person had good posture. Notice how the older woman uses the seat to support a healthy pelvic position while the younger woman tucks her pelvis in spite of the fine contours of the seat.

fig.F-20

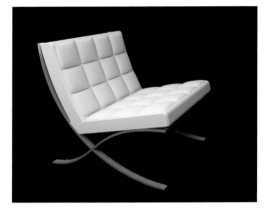

The Mies van der Rohe chair, first exhibited at the World Fair in Barcelona in 1929, reflects and perpetuates the trend of its day, forcing a tucked pelvis in the name of casual comfort.

THE EFFECT ON OUR BACKS

Whatever the cause, many of us are faced with the reality of a distorted and compressed spinal column. This may be fairly benign, but it usually gets worse over decades until the cumulative compression crosses a threshold. Beyond that threshold lies the potential for real damage to nerves, bones, and discs, with accompanying pain. Sometimes the pain does not arise directly from the damaged tissues, but rather from muscle spasms in the back that are a protective response to the worsening situation. Pain, whether from damage or muscle spasms, is what drives most patients to seek relief. It is very likely why you are reading this book.

I have dealt with back problems for more than 30 years and only wish I had met Esther Gokhale much earlier. In spite of trying various conventional and alternative treatments including surgery, I had constant background pain and many, many days of being debilitated. Esther was the first person who really helped me. Her posture method has been invaluable.

Mark Tuschman, photographer,
Menlo Park, CA

MOVING OUT OF MISERY

In your efforts to reduce or eliminate your back pain, you may have tried well-established interventions that physicians typically recommend: anti-inflammatories, muscle relaxants, physical therapy, injections, and even surgery. You may also have tried such alternative therapies as chiropractic, acupuncture, massage, yoga, or the host of specialized techniques popular today.

At last you have come to the right place! By re-establishing natural posture and movement patterns, you will be addressing the root cause of your pain, regaining and maintaining a pain-free back.

As you learn my technique, you can also expect it to:

• Reduce or eliminate other muscle and joint pain
• Prevent further muscle and joint degeneration and injury
• Increase your energy, stamina, and flexibility
• Reduce stress and improve your appearance

As you will discover, my method is quick to learn and effective from the beginning. Equipment needs are limited to a good chair, a few cushions, and good shoes. Once you have learned the key principles, the method puts almost no demands on your time. You integrate the basic principles into all your positions and movements, and your physical activities become effective exercises to stretch and strengthen your body, rather than hurt it (fig.F-21).

HOW IT WORKS

You will learn to sit, sleep, stand, walk, and bend in ways that protect and strengthen your bones and muscles, in ways for which the body was designed.

• Sitting will be comfortable, either with a backrest when you place your back in therapeutic traction (stretchsitting) or without a backrest, when you stack your spine on a well-positioned, *anteverted* pelvis (stacksitting).
• Sleeping will be comfortable and provide hours of restorative traction, whether lying on your back or side (stretchlying).
• Standing will be a resting position for most of the muscles of the body with the weight-bearing bones vertically stacked over the heels (tallstanding).

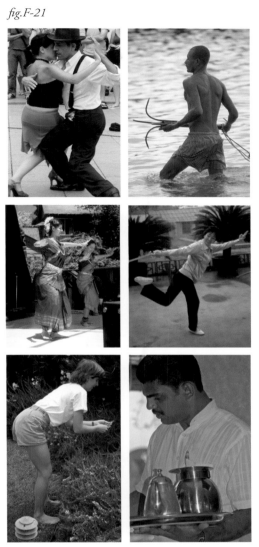

fig.F-21

Everyday movements serve as therapeutic stretching or strengthening exercises.

• Bending will involve hinging at the hip rather than the waist, exercising the long back muscles and sparing the spinal discs and ligaments (hip-hinging).
• Actions that challenge spinal structures, such as carrying or twisting, will use particular muscles of the abdomen and back (inner corset) to protect the spine.
• Walking will be a series of smooth forward propulsions, challenging the muscles of the lower body and sparing the weight-bearing joints throughout the body (glidewalking).

In relearning these everyday actions, you will reposition and reshape your shoulders, arms, neck, torso, hips, legs, and feet the way they were designed to be. You will develop a high level of confidence in and sense of control over your well-being.

- Because of the emphasis on lengthening and decompressing the spine, you will remove some of the stresses that cause disc degeneration and certain arthritic changes.

- Because you will spend so many hours a day decompressing your spine through gentle "traction," you may regain as much as an inch in height.

- Because of the emphasis on correct stacking and alignment, you will increase the deposition of bone where needed and help to prevent osteoporosis.

- Because your muscles can relax at rest, your circulation will improve. This enables your system to efficiently nourish and heal your tissues and clear waste products.

- Because of altered alignment, your breathing mechanism will change, with more action in the rib cage. Over time, this enlarges the rib cage and allows for greater lung capacity, improved processing of oxygen, and extra energy.

- Because you are using your muscles and sparing your joints, you will be less prone to injury and joint degeneration.

The posture work that I have done with Esther has made a dramatic impact on my quality of life. For more than 10 years, I had suffered from chronic back problems. Until I worked with Esther, my back was a near constant source of pain and I was guaranteed to have a couple of major "episodes" every year that severely limited my mobility for at least a week per episode. Since working with Esther, I have become generally pain free and have been episode-free for more than 18 months: and I now measure 1/2 inch taller than before, thanks to my newfound posture. The work has led me to feel better and have more confidence.

Edward Spiegel, Palo Alto, CA

WHAT DOES GOOD POSTURE LOOK LIKE?

If you lived a hundred years ago or in a village in Portugal or Africa today, you would have a good sense of what healthy posture looks like. Since you live in a modern industrialized society, and are surrounded by people who have poor posture, it is helpful to articulate some of the characteristics that constitute good posture. Refer to figs.F-22,23 as you read the following description.

The pelvis is tipped forward or anteverted. An easy way to see this is to imagine a belt line and notice that it angles downward toward the front. Pelvic anteversion is accompanied by a pronounced angle low in the spine (between the L5 and S1 vertebrae), the lumbo-sacral arch. This is distinct from a swayback, which occurs higher in the upper lumbar spine.

There is an even groove over the vertical midline of the back. The groove is not especially deep in any location (for example, the low back), nor are the vertebrae prominent in any location (for example, the upper back). The entire spine above the lumbo-sacral arch has relatively little curvature.

The shoulders are positioned posteriorly relative to the torso, with the result that the arms align with the back of the torso. The arms are somewhat externally rotated so that the thumbs, or even the palms, face forward.

The front contour of the torso is dome-like and smooth. The lower border of the rib cage does not protrude from, but rather is flush with, the abdominal contour. The chest is full with a raised sternum as a result of the chest expanding with every breath.

There is a soft angle at the groin between the front of the torso and the legs that permits the femoral arteries, veins, and nerves to function without compromise.

The chin, and an imaginary line joining the middle of the ear and the tip of the nose, angle downward as a result of a relaxed and elongated cervical spine.

The buttock muscles are well developed because they are in a position of mechanical advantage and are used in walking.

The muscles throughout the body have good tone (not bunched up with long taut tendons attached to bone).

fig. F-22

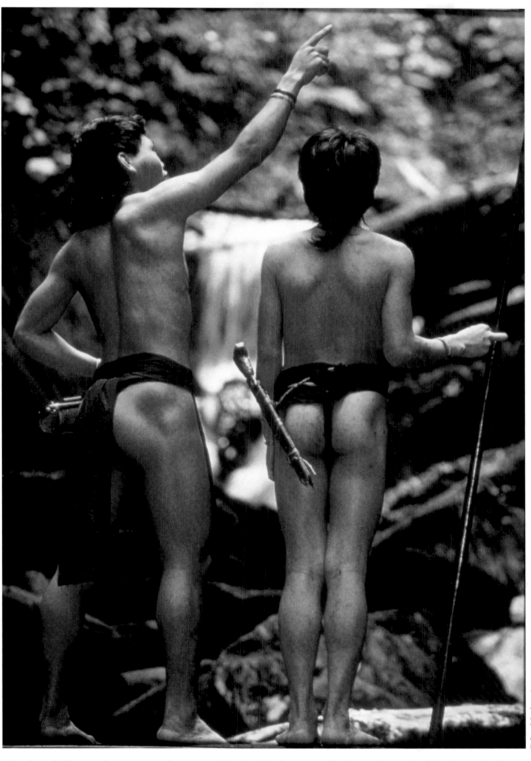

© Ian Mackenzie

This duo of Ubong tribesmen was photographed by Ian Mackenzie (published in Nomads of the Dawn*). He generously agreed to let me use the photograph which, more than any other, lives in my mind's eye and reminds me of the beauty, strength, and grace that is natural to our species. Notice that the buttocks are positioned well behind the spine and are well-developed, the shoulder blades are also positioned behind the spine, the groove over the midline of the back is even, the feet point slightly outward and have well-developed arches, and the muscles in general are toned but not taut.*

The main weight-bearing bones in the body are vertically aligned over the heels.

The feet point 10-15 degrees outwards and the arches of the foot are muscular and pronounced.

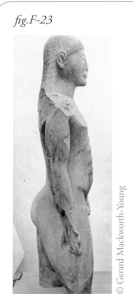

fig.F-23

In this Greek statue, notice the pronounced lumbo-sacral angle and the relatively flat upper lumbar spine, the arm hanging along the back of the torso, the chin angled down, the lower border of the rib cage flush with the front contour of the torso, and the soft angle at the groin.

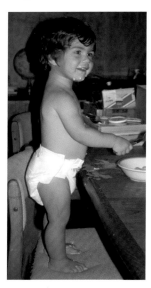

In my year-old daughter, notice the pronounced lumbo-sacral angle and the relatively flat upper lumbar spine, the chin angled down, the soft angle at the groin, and the vertebrae and leg bones stacked over the heels.

ANTEVERTED PELVIS

Pelvic anteversion is the foundation of a healthy human frame, affecting the placement of every other part of the body.

Today, many medical and fitness experts advise a "neutral" pelvic position that is slightly (and sometimes extremely) tucked, or *retroverted* [26]. A retroverted pelvis leads you into one of two postures: you can be upright, but your low back muscles will be tense; or you can relax, but your upper body will slump forward (fig.F-24b,c). Neither of these postures is healthy; both cause damage.

In this book, you will learn how to position your pelvis in the natural way seen in babies, indigenous peoples, and your ancestors. The ideal position is one of significant forward tilt or anteversion (fig.F-24a). This will allow for natural stacking of the vertebrae without muscle strain and good alignment of the spine over the leg bones. The weight-bearing bones in the body get the healthy level of stress they need (to prevent osteoporosis), and the muscles get the relaxation they need. It also puts your leg and buttock muscles in a position of mechanical advantage.

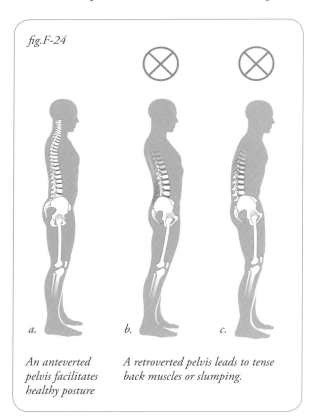

fig.F-24

a.   *b.*   *c.*

An anteverted pelvis facilitates healthy posture

A retroverted pelvis leads to tense back muscles or slumping.

When we evolved from being quadrupedal to bipedal, the L5-S1 disc became wedge-shaped. Anteverting the pelvis preserves the wedge-shaped space that accommodates this disc perfectly (fig. F-25a). Any other pelvic position compromises the L5-S1 disc. Retroversion puts pressure on the anterior part of the disc, forcing the contents toward the posterior and wearing its fibrous exterior (fig. F-25b). Disc damage ranges from *bulging* to *herniation* to *sequestration*.

Note that a lumbo-sacral angle is different from a sway back. The lumbo-sacral angle is a natural curve very low in the spine (between L5 and S1); a sway is an unhealthy curve higher up in the lumbar spine.

In addition to affecting the bones, spinal discs, and muscles, the position of the pelvis also affects the pelvic organs. An anteverted pelvis allows for ample space in the pelvic cavity and optimal circulation in the pelvic organs; a retroverted pelvis compresses the pelvic organs into an unnaturally small space, compromising their shape, orientation, and function. On learning to antevert their pelvis, many of my patients report improvement in conditions such as irritable bowel syndrome and constipation, menstrual irregularities like painful cramps and bloating (in women), prostate problems (in men), and fertility issues. I look forward to research studies done in these areas.

An anteverted pelvis places the pubic bone directly under the pelvic organs, providing a strong bony support beneath them; a retroverted pelvis leaves all such support to the rather flimsy Kegel (*pubo-coccygeal*) muscle (fig. 3-9 on page 73). In my clinical experience, a tucked (retroverted) pelvis predisposes women for organ prolapse and urinary incontinence; restoring pelvic anteversion helps with these conditions if they are not too advanced. Again, a research study in this area would be valuable.

Since the hamstring muscles attach to the sitz bones (*ischial tuberosities*), a retroverted pelvis permits the hamstring muscles to adapt to a shorter than normal resting length. This increases their susceptibility to injury. Anteversion maintains a healthy baseline length in the hamstrings, thus protecting them against injury.

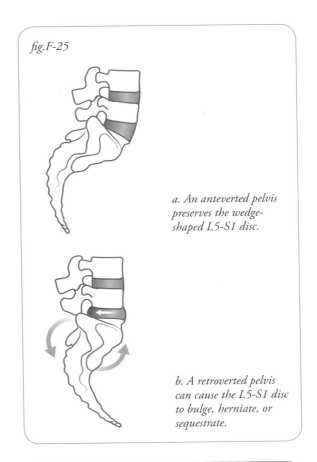

fig.F-25

a. An anteverted pelvis preserves the wedge-shaped L5-S1 disc.

b. A retroverted pelvis can cause the L5-S1 disc to bulge, herniate, or sequestrate.

I... believe my changed posture has affected the workings of my intestines. I used to stand with my stomach tight, my cheeks tucked under, and ribs high. As a runner I run very relaxed and on long runs I would suddenly have to move my bowels; to be more accurate, they would just suddenly want to move and I was in trouble! Now on long runs I have no problem. I guess it is because now my belly is always relaxed, so when I run there isn't a big change for my intestines.

Rita Czamanske, Masters runner, Palo Alto, CA

A GENTLY CURVED, ELONGATED SPINE

The ideal shape of the spine is a gentle, elongated curve, not an exaggerated "S" curve. Pronounced curvature should occur only at L5-S1 at the base of the spine.

In current lay and medical thinking, a normal spine curves significantly forward in the low back (lumbar spine), backward in the upper back (thoracic spine) and forward again in the neck (cervical spine). "Chin up and chest out," a directive many people follow when trying to have "good posture," results in exaggerated spinal curves. A lot of modern furniture and clothing reflects and perpetuates exaggerated spinal curvature. Lumbar cushions and cervical pillows, for example, are designed to support and even create these "natural" curves.

Medical literature, on the other hand, establishes that reducing spinal curvature can alleviate compression, reduce pain, and increase comfort.[27,28] Though most research on curvature in the lumbar area does not distinguish between lower and upper lumbar curvature, one paper reports on the radiographic examinations of upper and lower lumbar curvature in subjects with and without low back pain. The results are consistent with my claims: the back pain patients had more upper lumbar curvature and less lower lumbar curvature, whereas the subjects without pain had more lower lumbar curvature and less upper.[29]

> *I wouldn't have thought that at age 40 you could actually reverse curvature in the spine. Now I have no pain at all and I can do all sorts of exercise without getting injured.*
>
> Manda Mafy, Marketing Manager, Silicon Graphics, Mountain View, CA

> *I am surprised and pleased that I have been able to get rid of my dowager's hump by using techniques I learned from this method.*
>
> Anne White, Trager therapist, Davidson, NC

> *Esther's posture work has given me relief from chronic neck pain that physical therapy was unable to address. I am now pain-free even when sitting for long periods or flying long distances.*
>
> Dan Leemon, Chief Strategy Officer, Charles Schwab & Co., San Francisco, CA

EVERY BONE IN ITS NATURAL PLACE

The particular arrangement of the human skeleton is a product of the demands of upright living and the constant force of gravity over the span of human existence. Each bone has a natural place relative to its neighbors. Adjacent bones are designed to fit together in a certain way.

Our weight-bearing bones need stress to remain strong. Without this stress, calcium leaches from the bones or is inadequately deposited, leading to osteopenia and osteoporosis. Weight-bearing exercise provides the healthy stress that keeps bones strong. However, stress on the wrong part of the bone, caused by misalignment, can lead to arthritic changes such as bone spurs (*osteophytes*).

In this book, you will learn how to restore your bones to their proper places, reducing harmful stress while restoring healthy stress in the bones.

Our spines are not the only bony structures that suffer from misalignment. Our feet, knees, and hips are also subject to problems from poor alignment.

Foot problems

When we evolved from being quadrupedal to bipedal, the heel became reinforced to bear most of the weight of our upright structure. By comparison, the bones in the front of the foot are delicate. Today, instead of carrying most of the weight on their heels, many people displace their weight forward to the middle or front of the foot, putting undue stress on bones that are not designed to bear such weight. Doing so increases the chances of having bunions, sesamoid bone fractures, and plantar fasciitis.

Knee problems

Rotating the knees inward, a common problem, correlates with pronation of the foot and under-use of the buttock muscles. If the legs are misaligned as they bear the body's weight, they are subject to increased wear and tear, especially when bending, and make the knee joint more prone to injury. Rotating the knees inward increases the chances of torn ligaments, frayed menisci, and arthritic changes in the knee.

Another common knee problem is hyperextension or "locking the knees." Locked knees are a classic element of poor posture, causing muscles to be tense and inhibiting good circulation. Locked knees are usually accompanied by improper hip position, which has its own set of problems.

Hip problems

In our culture it is rare to find good alignment in the hip joint. People tend to "park" their hips forward, significantly misaligning the head of the femur in the hip socket (*acetabulum*). The muscles that bridge the area become tense in this misalignment. This tension reduces the natural gap between the ball and socket and can result in bone-to-bone contact. Over time, the unnatural stresses can lead to arthritic changes and possibly even the need for hip replacement surgery.

Hip misalignment can also occlude the femoral arteries, veins, and nerves, affecting circulation to and from the legs and feet. Symptoms of this condition include cold feet, Raynaud's Syndrome, and slowed healing of leg injuries.

In the "Tallstanding" lesson, you will learn the natural alignment of your pelvis on the heads of the femurs. In the "Glidewalking" lesson, you will learn to reestablish the natural gap between the head of the femur and hip socket (*acetabulum*).

USING MUSCLES MORE THAN JOINTS

In many daily activities, people under-use their muscles and overuse their joints. This has a doubly negative effect: muscles do not get enough healthy stress to remain strong; joints get too much stress, leading to wear and tear. For example, walking poorly, as most people do, is hard on the weight-bearing joints of the knees, hips, and spine, and jolts the frame with every step. It may also leave the buttock and leg muscles underused. As you will learn in this book, walking well uses muscles in the legs and buttocks to propel the body forward smoothly to a soft landing, sparing the joints from the stress of significant impact. The muscles gain strength; the joints remain undamaged.

You will also learn how to bend in a way that uses your muscles more and your joints less. Bending poorly is hard on the spinal discs and ligaments, and leaves the muscles of the back largely unchallenged. On the other hand, bending well engages the long muscles of the back and spares the spinal discs and ligaments. Again, muscles gain strength while joints remain healthy.

In Lesson 5, you will learn to use your "inner corset" in the face of threatened spinal compression or distortion. Again, this is a technique that takes the burden off the joints (the spinal discs), where it would be harmful, and puts it on the muscles (abdominal and intrinsic back muscles), where it is beneficial.

MUSCLES FULLY RELAXED WHEN NOT WORKING

When something goes wrong with our musculo-skeletal systems, we are often directed to muscle-strengthening exercises as a solution (as in most physical therapy regimens). While we are keenly aware of the need for muscle strength, we may not adequately appreciate the importance of muscle relaxation.

To maintain strength, a muscle must be allowed to relax. Thorough muscle relaxation facilitates good circulation, delivering nutrients and clearing waste products. Many people spend hours tensing their muscles unnecessarily. Often the tension is initiated through poor alignment; then it becomes habit. Reorganizing skeletal structures can break the cycle, enabling muscles to be relaxed when appropriate and to be tense only when needed.

BREATHING AS A THERAPEUTIC EXERCISE

Breathing does more than oxygenate the system. The physical action of breathing has its own therapeutic value: it exercises the key tissues of the chest and spinal area, keeping the area well circulated and healthy. Breathing is nature's way of exercising the area around your spine even when you are not engaged in aerobic activity. The natural elastic movement of every breath includes a mild lengthening of the spine with every inhalation and a settling back with every exhalation, and provides a gentle massage-like action that stimulates good circulation to support healthy tissues 24 hours a day.

As your vertebrae become better stacked, the muscles around your spine will relax, which will facilitate the elastic action of breathing. The chest and spine move the most during breathing at rest; the diaphragm and abdomen become more involved when exercise or other activities place a greater demand on the lungs. In general, you will find that as your posture improves, your muscles will relax and your lung capacity will increase.

> *When you've been ill for a long time, you have a chance to try out a lot of stuff. This work really stands out. It makes a difference in how you breathe, and a lot of improvements follow from that.*
>
> Robin Pfaff, business owner,
> Palo Alto, CA

IT WORKS!

Nearly all my patients improve, many with profound and far-reaching results. Even patients with a long history of pain, who have become skeptical about their chances of improvement, often find a solution. They no longer depend on pain medication. They're relieved to have avoided surgery. They feel in control because they understand what caused their pain and they know how to prevent it. Here are a few testimonials:

I have had significant problems with low back pain and sciatica for more than two decades. At several points I was unable to walk more than fifty yards without squatting to relieve the pain, and required one back surgery for a slipped disc. Back pain often kept me from sleeping. I tried exercises and painkillers with mixed and generally poor results.

The person who has helped me the most over the years is Esther Gokhale. My back problem is now essentially under control. I no longer regularly wake up with a sore back and generally am able to walk five or more miles a day with little or no discomfort. If I avoid cramped long-term sitting (in a car or long tourist-class airline flight), I can mostly forget about the back that plagued me for so long.

The Gokhale Method℠ is logically based, compelling, and expertly delivered. It is unlike physical therapy and provides insights that should be more commonly available to back pain patients. I would like to see this approach become a part of standard care. Early access to this kind of intervention could have saved me a lot of pain and grief.

Paul Ehrlich, Professor of Biological Sciences
President, Center for Conservation Biology
Department of Biological Sciences,
Stanford University, Stanford, CA

I had been dancing professionally for only a little over three years when, in a New York ballet studio in 1989, I first strained my lower back. I had no idea at the time that this early, slight, seemingly innocuous injury was to lead, over the next thirteen years, to a long chain of back and neck injuries. These injuries grew – in a way which seemed, increasingly, to be nothing less than inexorable – in frequency and severity and duration.

Over the course of the following years I diligently – and with increasing pessimism and a growing sense of powerlessness – sought treatment from both traditional and non-traditional clinicians: I consulted several doctors (including surgeons and a prominent sports medicine specialist) and completed courses of treatment by two highly regarded physiotherapists; three chiropractors; an acupuncturist and Chinese herbalist; a number of massage and shiatsu practitioners; two yoga teachers specializing in back care; and specialists in a range of body therapies including (among others) the Alexander Technique, Feldenkrais Method, Applied Kinesiology, and Body Mind Centering.

These efforts met with little success, and I eventually became convinced that I was living with a chronic, degenerative – and essentially untreatable – back problem. I stopped dancing in 1991 and, over the course of the 1990s, experienced a gradual yet quite dramatic decrease in mobility. Once extremely physically active (dancing, practicing yoga and martial arts, running, swimming, hiking or working out with weights on a daily basis), I saw a radical reduction in the scope of what I could safely do with my body, eliminating first dance, then weight training, then yoga, then swimming in an attempt to control my back pain. By the year 2000 the only exercise that seemed not to exacerbate my back pain was walking. When I began learning the Gokhale Method℠ in 2002, I hadn't experienced a day or a night without pain in over a decade.

Through this method I learned healthy ways to sit, stand, lie, and walk, gradually adding a program of stretching, yoga poses, and exercises distilled from Indian and Brazilian dance. The positive effects were dramatic: Within weeks, my pain began to decrease. My mobility (as well as my optimism and general vitality) increased and, over a six-month period, I began yoga, weight training, swimming and – miraculously – dance. Today I am virtually pain free, and I am once again leading a physically exuberant life.

The Gokhale Method℠ brilliantly integrates a strong foundation in anatomy and physiology with elements of Chinese medicine, and the carefully researched study of movement and postural patterns from diverse regions. The method is both down-to-earth and elegant, and has helped me in ways I could not even have imagined. What I owe Esther Gokhale is inestimable: After years of unsuccessful attempts to address my chronic pain, I now have mobility, freedom. I cannot recommend this program more highly.

Ben Davidson, Ph.D., Assistant Dean of Students,
Stanford University, Stanford, CA

I became a patient of Esther Gokhale's in January 2004. I am grateful to Esther for leading me to a major improvement in the quality of my life by eliminating incapacitating bouts of lower back pain.

I felt immediate improvements after my first Gokhale Method℠ lesson, during which I learned how to put my lower back into traction while in bed. After a week, I was waking without the usual morning back stiffness. Similar instructions on how to arrange my back while driving were easy to implement and had an almost immediate payoff in functionality (being able to drive for an hour without emerging a listing wreck). Benefits continued as I learned subtleties of posture, breathing, stance, and walking. At the same time, my core muscles grew in strength to support my lower back.

One of the reasons the method works well is that all the positioning, strengthening, and stretching are done in the course of everyday activities: sitting at a desk, driving a car, weeding, walking. So, as opposed to the sets of crunches, pelvic tilts, and stretches the physical therapists advocated, I actually did the work, frequently. Additionally, the work produced an immediate improvement in how my back felt, as I did it, creating an incentive to continue. In other words, it was easy to remember to do the work because it automatically came to mind when my back was most likely to give me trouble. The work did not put any stress on my back, so it felt comfortable and safe, in contrast to my experience with physical therapy, in which some sets of exercises often increased the discomfort (and in one case caused me to re-injure my back).

Prior to my first visit with Esther, I had seen an orthopedist, a physiatrist, and a podiatrist; I had taken a lower-back training class and a course of physical therapy; I had tried a variety of anti-inflammatory, muscle-relaxant, and pain medications. I experienced constant low-grade pain. Yet an MRI showed no more than the wear and tear one might expect of a middle-aged woman who had spent too much of her youth carrying heavy backpacks full of rock samples.

In the five years prior to working with Esther, I spent several days in bed each year due to severe back pain, followed by intervals in which my mobility was greatly impaired and I had difficulty doing my job as a professor, traveling to professional meetings, or doing geologic fieldwork. Since first starting to learn the Gokhale Method℠, I have not had any serious back incidents. It is gratifying that, when I do get a little twinge, I have the skills to keep it from escalating into something incapacitating. I haven't missed any work; I have not needed codeine for pain; and I was able to compete in the U.S. nationals in dog agility (my hobby) in November 2004. This constitutes a significant improvement in the quality of my life. I still find it surprising that such a big improvement can be produced by such seemingly small adjustments that have no downside risk. A quantitative measure of my improvement is my height, which increased by 3/8" over the past year, placing me just shy of my youthful height.

Gail Mahood, Professor of Geology,
Stanford University, Stanford, CA

I had the good fortune to be referred to Esther Gokhale for help in rectifying a significant distortion of my posture and a severe limitation in my walking due to spinal stenosis and a broken-off fragment of inter-vertebral cartilage which impinged on a sciatic nerve. Since starting to work with Ms. Gokhale over one and a half years ago, I've taken no non-steroidal analgesics (previously I would have several episodes a month in which some were necessary), have received non-solicited spontaneous comments from friends and family on the improvement in my posture, and have resumed walks of some duration…It's a pleasure to be able to give her an unqualified endorsement

Milton Lozoff, MD,
Palo Alto, CA

Changing my posture changed my life. Thanks to this method, I am now free of the debilitating back pain that had plagued me since my adolescence.

Suzanne Hecker, Geologist, U.S. Geological Survey,
Menlo Park, CA

I was fascinated by how Esther Gokhale's method filled important gaps in my "dancer's placement." I got rid of my chronic neck pain and had loads of fun while getting the work done.

Julie Dorsey, former ballet dancer and teacher,
Atherton, CA

To read more remarks and letters from students, visit www.egwellness.com.

ORIENTATION

How to use the lessons

My husband had hunched posture as a teenager and into his twenties. He developed an interest in my work and attended classes occasionally over the years, resulting in some profound changes in his appearance and muscle health. On the left he is 28 years old; on the right he is 48.

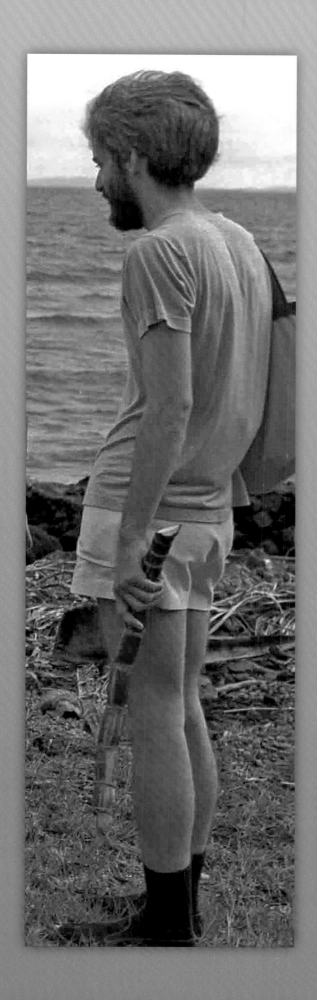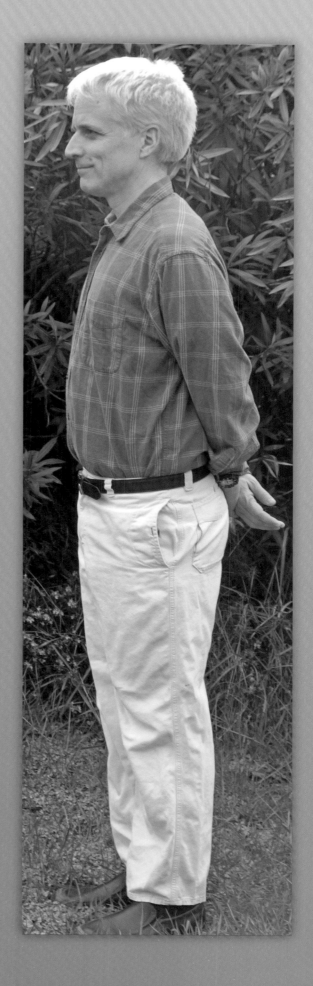

People can learn Gokhale Method℠ 101 by completing the lessons in the following chapters of the book. The lessons combine background information, supporting visuals, and precise step-by-step instructions. Just as a travel guide can lead you safely through the byways of a foreign city to introduce new sights and sounds, this book can guide you safely through the route to acquire improved, more healthful posture and ways of moving.

FOLLOW THE LESSON SEQUENCE

People new to my technique may feel a natural impatience to skip or hurry through some lessons and proceed to those that seem to address their area of concern. Based on my experience teaching this technique for 15 years, I encourage you to follow the lessons in sequence. By doing this, you should:

- Realize substantial postural improvement with the very first lesson, easing the pain and discomfort you may be experiencing
- Learn to support and protect delicate structures, ensuring that you can learn each technique safely
- Build skills in early lessons that are used in later ones, reducing the effort required to master the more complex skills

I encourage you to trust that the seemingly disparate parts within and across lessons will soon connect. Performing an architectural remodel of your frame is much like working a puzzle: most of the time, you work on isolated areas, not necessarily seeing how they will later fit together. For example, for most people it is not apparent that working on foot position will help resolve back pain. Because it is important occasionally to see the big picture, I have included explanations with each lesson to help provide that overview.

Some situations require that you modify your route through this material. The following are exceptions to the recommendation that you complete the lessons in sequence.

HERNIATED DISC
Caution:
If you have a diagnosis, or any suspicion, of a herniated disc in the lower lumbar area, you should be working with a medical professional as you learn the techniques in this book. It is extremely important that you not proceed to Lessons 3 (Stacksitting), 4 (Stretchlying on Your Side), and 7 (Hip-hinging) until you have mastered the ability to maintain extra length at the site of

the injury. Gaining additional length in the back is therapeutic and safe for everyone. Lessons 1, 2, and 5 teach you to lengthen your spine, which will make you more comfortable and can accelerate healing of the injured disc. The recommended lesson sequence, then, is 1, 2, 5, 6, 8. From Appendix 1, focus especially on the exercises for strengthening the muscles of the torso.

HIGH IMPACT ACTIVITIES
Activities that involve high impact (such as running or impact aerobics), if done incorrectly, carry a significant risk of damage to spinal discs. If you participate in such activities, you may want to begin immediately to protect your back. I recommend you read over Lesson 5 (Using Your Inner Corset). You will gain insights that have immediate value, although you will understand them better after having completed Lessons 1-4.

BENDING ACTIVITIES
If your everyday activities involve a lot of bending (for example, gardening), be aware that, of all actions, bending technique correlates most closely with back health. People who bend well usually enjoy good back health; people who bend poorly often develop back pain. If currently you have no back pain, read Lesson 7 (Hip-hinging) to begin exploring a better way to bend. (Stop if you experience any discomfort.) Then proceed through the lessons in their normal sequence. When you encounter the bending lesson a second time, you will refine your technique and transform your bending activities into healthy exercise.

ALLOW TIME TO CHANGE

People often ask how long it will take to learn this technique. There is no pat answer to that question. Changing the way we move requires re-patterning the brain, as it discards an old set of habits and replaces it with a new one. We need to "rewire" how we sit, lie, stand, and move, changing these basic movements. People learn at different speeds.

In general, a person who is engaged in a variety of physical activities and sports tends to readily absorb new kinesthetic input. Yet sometimes very sedentary people surprise me with their kinesthetic acuity for this particular training. These people may experience quick success because the training is so basic. And sometimes a person with extensive physical training must work hard to unlearn certain ingrained ways. However, most people are pleasantly surprised at how quickly they learn this technique. Perhaps it is because they are returning to a more natural way of moving, one that was familiar to them in their early years. As they relearn these forgotten habits, the "new" ways of sitting, lying, and moving become natural and automatic.

As with any physical transition, you might experience some initial difficulty. While you are learning a new posture or way of moving, be sure to explore the change gradually. Don't force your body to achieve the ideal result immediately, as that may strain your muscles. Instead, let your body gradually adapt to the ideal over time.

Common wisdom holds that you must repeat an action at least 20 times for it to become habit. Be patient as you work to integrate the techniques into your daily movements. You will create these new habits more from a sustained awareness over time than from an infrequent but heroic effort. The only requirement is that you not let your awareness slip away.

KNOW WHAT TO EXPECT

HOW QUICKLY CAN I EXPECT RESULTS?
Most people enjoy immediate benefits from the very first lesson, in which they learn the technique of "stretchsitting" to lengthen the spine. Not only is this the safest posture modification for a compromised spine, it also is simple to understand and easy to execute. Some of the subsequent lessons may take a bit longer, but should provide tangible benefits.

The method blends intellectual, visual, and kinesthetic cues. As you learn each new postural shift, you will simultaneously understand it, see it, and feel it. Because the learning occurs on three levels, it accelerates and deepens the process of turning these shifts into new habits.

HOW LONG SHOULD EACH LESSON TAKE?
Hurrying through the lessons offers no advantage and, in fact, reduces your chances of success. You should expect to spend 15 to 45 minutes on each new lesson. Subsequently, as you integrate the material into your daily activities, it will take a few seconds each time. For example, when you first seat yourself at your desk or in your car, you should concentrate on the fine points of positioning yourself well. Then forget about your posture and enjoy a period of relaxation, allowing your body to gain muscle memory from this pose.

Allow enough time between lessons so that you can incorporate your new learning into your everyday life, as your brain re-patterns each new physical skill. It is possible to do up to two lessons per day (our accelerated program, taken mostly by people from out-of-town, includes one or two lessons each day), but many people prefer a lesson a week.

HOW DIFFICULT ARE THE LESSONS?
Although the steps in each lesson are simple, they are not necessarily easy. Certain steps tend to be difficult for everybody; other steps are easy for some people and hard for others. Sometimes the difficulties are caused by physical limitations associated with age, pathology, or obesity. Sometimes the necessary re-patterning in the brain is extensive and therefore challenging. During the re-patterning, a particular position or movement may seem unnatural because it is not yet habit.

Learning new movement patterns is similar to learning a new language, which ideally alternates periods of immersion and usage with periods of attention to detail. In learning the language of movement, you will benefit from a mix of focusing on large-scale movements and on finer points.

> *The techniques are simple and can be learned by anyone.*
>
> Michael Smith, software engineer, Palo Alto, CA

UNDERSTAND HOW THE LESSONS ARE ORGANIZED

Each lesson is organized into three sections:
- An introduction provides background and discusses the importance of the posture or movement, describes its benefits, and includes specific caveats where necessary.
- Instructions provide detailed step-by-step instructions with accompanying photographs. Photographs marked with an ⊗ show what not to do. Page sidebars include lists of required equipment, anatomical drawings, and schematics to help you understand the material, and photos of good technique to inspire you.
- Wrap-up includes indications of improvement, troubleshooting, further information, and a lesson recap.

RECOGNIZE YOUR PROGRESS

When learning any new skill, you will move through four stages of mastery. As you are working on a new posture or movement, try to recognize the stage you are in.

STAGE 1
UNDERSTANDING THE MOVEMENTS INTELLECTUALLY

Each lesson teaches a posture or movement through discussion and demonstration. By carefully reading and studying the material, you should be able to achieve Stage 1.

> *The fact that the student is asked to think about the problem and is made a part of the treatment process is, in my mind, the strongest part of the program. Rather than adopting a particular regime for solving a problem, the student is encouraged to experiment with and think about the problem, using the tools provided by the program. This was the key for me, and I think it can be the key for many other people as well.*
>
> Gunnar Carlsson, Professor, Department of Mathematics, Stanford University, CA

STAGE 2
PERFORMING THE MOVEMENTS WITH GUIDANCE

Using each lesson as your guide, you should be able to imitate the posture or movement. Remember that you may be unable to achieve the ideal result at first, but you should work to approximate it.

STAGE 3
PERFORMING THE MOVEMENTS WITHOUT GUIDANCE

Stage 3 is the ability to step yourself through the process of sitting, lying, or moving without referring to the lesson. You should be able to remember the steps to position your body appropriately.

STAGE 4
PERFORMING THE MOVEMENTS WITHOUT CONSCIOUS AWARENESS

This is, of course, the goal of your training, and may take some time. Regular practice (Stage 3) is the secret to reaching this stage. Eventually, you will have moments of awareness when you realize you are indeed using the technique but have not used conscious thought to do so.

GENERAL HEALTH IMPROVEMENT

In addition to reducing or eliminating back pain, most students experience other health improvements. These may be physical, physiological, or psychological. Students over the years have reported improvements in muscle and joint problems, sleep, digestion, respiration, menstrual ease (women), urinary function, sex drive, mood, energy level, self-esteem, and athletic performance.

> *I have been able to rid myself of carpal tunnel syndrome by using this method. It was a very pleasant process—Every session was like a mini-vacation.*
>
> Kate Orrange, computer worker, San Mateo, CA

> *I was amazed to learn how differently I could feel by making basic changes in the way I sat, stood, and breathed.*
>
> Jane Battaglia, acupuncturist, Berkeley, CA

BARRIERS TO SUCCESS

MUSCLE SORENESS

Be aware that you might experience some muscle soreness as you transform your posture. Underused muscles may complain at their new, more demanding role. Surprisingly, overused muscles that now relax may also cause some discomfort, due to the release of lactic acid into the surrounding tissue. In both cases, this soreness is temporary and can be relieved by hot baths, massage, rest, or acupuncture. Take a little more time with the lessons, be careful as you practice new techniques, and soon the soreness will pass.

"IT FEELS WEIRD"

At first, you may feel awkward in these new poses and movements. Some people describe this feeling as "weird but comfortable." As the strangeness diminishes, many people report that the new ways now feel "right"; the old ways of moving no longer feel comfortable. What they are feeling is valid, in two senses. They are returning to kinesthetic ways that are genetically encoded, and that were natural in their early years before they learned our culture's bad habits.

"IT STILL HURTS"

The technique won't work if you just go through the lessons and forget about them. You need to apply what you learn to your everyday life and everyday movements. If you simply complete the lessons, but don't work to integrate what you've learned, you will easily slip back into your old habits – the ones that caused much of your back pain.

"MY CLOTHES DON'T FIT"

It would be unfair not to mention the only downside to learning this technique: over time your body shape may change enough that your more tailored clothing no longer fits. Current fashions are cut for today's average posture, which includes rounded shoulders and a tucked pelvis. Your new carriage may require you to alter or replace some of your fitted clothing. This seems a small price to pay for your improved health and appearance.

BACKSLIDING

Whenever you learn something new, there is a tendency to backslide to your old habits. In this case, the tendency is aggravated because you are surrounded by people with poor posture. We are natural mimics and unconsciously replicate the posture and movements we see. Therefore, after completing the lessons in this book, most people find it helpful to refresh their learning through a monthly maintenance activity. Here are some suggestions:

- Review the lessons you found most transforming, or the ones that gave you the most trouble.
- Tour a museum to observe and critique how artists have rendered human posture.
- Visit a culture with intact posture traditions.
- Do something that reinforces the technique you have learned, such as taking yoga or dance classes taught by an informed instructor, or practicing a sport with an informed coach. (Posture and movement training is not a substitute for physical activity; I encourage you to pursue your favorite activities, and incorporate the principles in this book.)
- Communicate with other people working on their posture (visit www.egwellness.com).

Readers living in or willing to visit the San Francisco Bay area have the option of refresher courses at the Esther Gokhale Wellness Center in Palo Alto. For more information, contact us at 650-324-3244 or info@egwellness.com.

Esther has the gift of suggestion. She is very subtle with her words and her hands. At times it almost felt to me as if Esther's subtle combination of images, phrases, and direct suggestions to the musculo-skeletal system operated subliminally to gently entice my body back into its ancestral posture.

Barbara Lane, housewife,
Palo Alto, CA

While working intensively on a book, I developed a version of repetitive stress syndrome that gradually made my hands and forearms virtually useless. I experienced intense burning and numbness, and ended up finishing the book (under a deadline) using my two index fingers. I saw several medical doctors, underwent physical therapy, wore various wrist devices, redesigned my writing places to be more ergonomic, took scheduled breaks from the computer, and so on... Nothing worked. After a matter of weeks of posture work, acupuncture and acupressure, I recovered the full use of my hands and forearms.

Gretchen C. Daily, Professor, Biological Sciences, Stanford University, CA

Esther Gokhale helped me resolve a five year injury after nothing else had worked. Her work is unique and thorough.

Patti Sue Plumer, lawyer/runner (World Record holder for 1500m and 500m run in 1992; three-time Olympian), Menlo Park, CA

1

STRETCHSITTING

Sitting with a lengthened back

This Burkina woman came to the village well with her baby to do her laundry. I was enchanted by her strength and grace. Here she is stretching her baby's back in a way similar to what you will learn in this lesson. The baby is in a period of rapid growth and benefits from the periodic stretch to his back muscles.

Notice that the mother's shoulders are positioned well back relative to her torso, her neck is elongated without significant curvature, her chin angles downwards, she positions her baby behind the middle of her body close to her spine, and she uses her forearm rather than her hand to support most of the baby's weight.

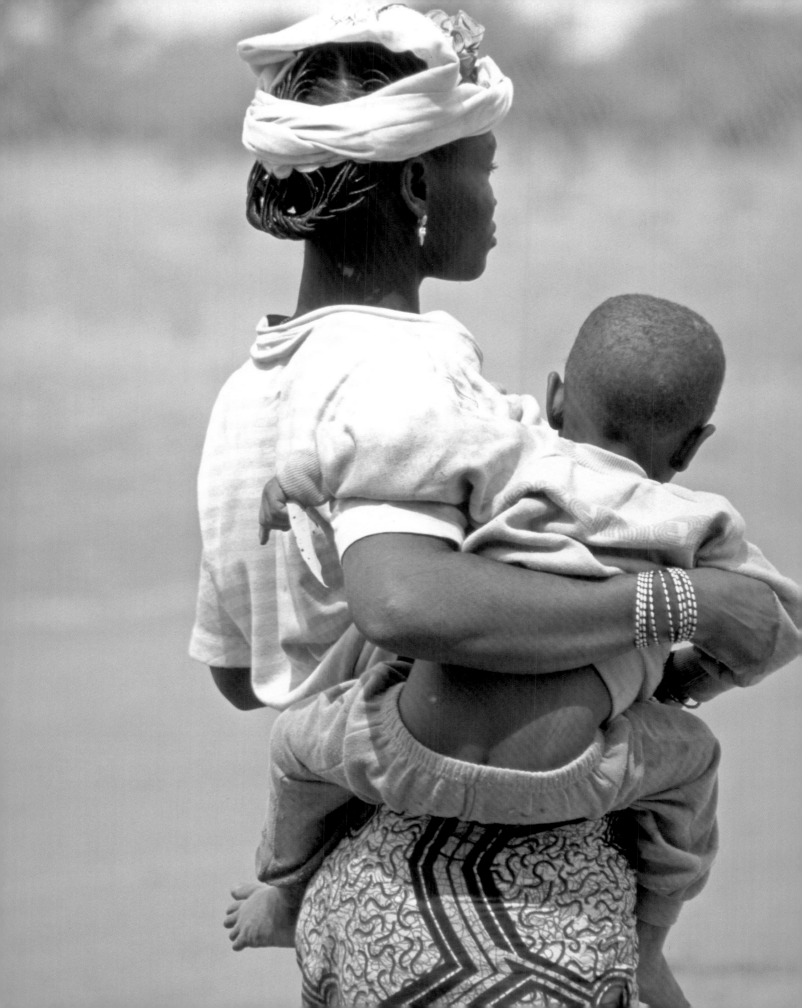

In this lesson, you will learn to put your back into gentle traction when seated, a technique I call "stretchsitting." This simple but powerful technique will not only give you a comfortable way to sit, but also help undo some of the damage caused by years of hunching (fig.1-1) or swaying (fig.1-2).

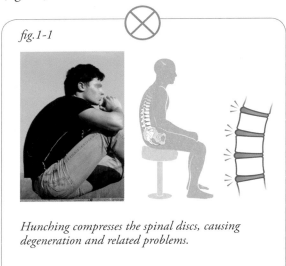

fig.1-1

Hunching compresses the spinal discs, causing degeneration and related problems.

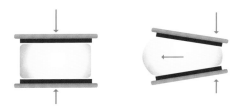

The effect of hunching is similar to what happens when pressure is applied to one side of 'Smores.

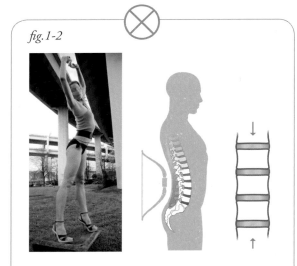

fig.1-2

Swaying arches the spine excessively, compresses the discs, and compromises circulation around the spine. The result is similar to a tightly strung bow.

When you stretchsit, you lengthen your spine against the back of a chair. This immediately decompresses your discs (fig.1-3), preventing further damage and allowing them to heal. The long muscles of your back get a significant and sustained stretch, helping them adjust to healthier, longer baseline lengths. Over a period of months, you can expect to become 1/4" to 1" taller, depending on how much height you have lost to extra curvature or compression in your spine. The additional length in your spine may also result in related health benefits, such as improved circulation and nerve function around the spine.

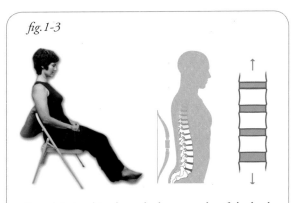

fig.1-3

Stretchsitting lengthens the long muscles of the back in an action similar to relaxing a bow. Stretchsitting also decompresses the discs, allowing them to heal and preventing further damage.

As part of stretchsitting, you will restore your shoulders to a natural baseline position by doing a "shoulder roll." This will augment the blood circulation to and from your arms, accelerating repair of any damaged tissue and preventing injury. If you have arm problems such as carpal tunnel syndrome or a repetitive stress injury, it is important that you learn to reposition your shoulders. Hunching your shoulders while placing demands on your arms, as when typing, playing a musical instrument, using a game console, or playing a racquet sport, is especially problematic (fig.1-4). While the activity increases the demand for blood, the compromised shoulder architecture reduces the supply. Positioning your shoulders well allows you to work and exercise longer without pain or injury (fig.1-5).

As part of stretchsitting, you will also learn to lengthen and align your neck. Not only will your neck feel more comfortable, but the nerves that emanate from your cervical spine will function

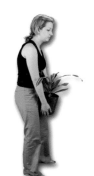
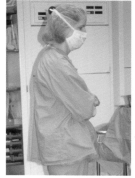

fig.1-4

Hunched shoulders compromise circulation to and from the arms and predispose people to injury.

Compression in the neck can result in cervical disc and nerve damage.

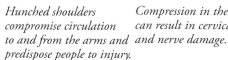

fig.1-5

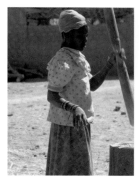
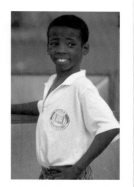

Well-aligned shoulders allow for good circulation to and from the arms, and protect against injury.

A well-aligned neck allows the cervical discs and nerves to remain healthy.

they already have the necessary length in their spines to optimize disc and nerve health (fig.1-8 on page 37).

Note some important differences between stretchsitting and other common ways of stretching the back:

- Stretchsitting is beneficial for muscles and discs alike; many conventional back stretches compromise the discs as they stretch the muscles (fig.1-6).
- Stretchsitting takes no time out of your schedule and yet provides hours of therapeutic effect; conventional back stretches take time and can realistically be done for only a few minutes a day.
- The cumulative benefits from stretchsitting are much more significant than those from back stretches.

There are several reasons why stretchsitting is the first technique you will learn. It is safe (if your back and neck muscles spasm easily, be sure to lengthen your spine very slowly and gently). It is easy to learn. It helps protect your spine from injury as you prepare for later lessons. And it should produce benefits immediately, especially if you have compression in your spine.

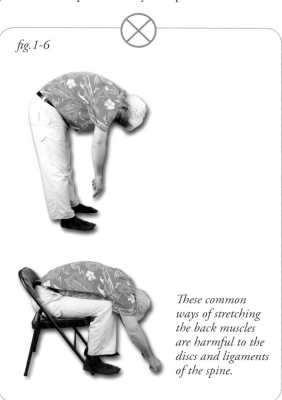

fig.1-6

These common ways of stretching the back muscles are harmful to the discs and ligaments of the spine.

better. If you have tingling or numbness down your arms, for example, the techniques taught here are crucial to your recovery. Since every nerve that distributes to the arms originates in the neck, restoring healthy neck architecture can help alleviate arm nerve problems.

In this lesson you will also learn the basics of healthy foot alignment. (Lesson 6 explains more about how foot shape relates to posture: the goal here is merely to gain familiarity with this new foot position.)

Stretchsitting may strike you as a little contrived. In a way, it is. People in traditional cultures do not need to actively stretchsit in this way because

BENEFITS

- Resets the baseline length of long back muscles, reducing muscle pain

- Decompresses the spinal discs, preventing further disc damage and reducing disc pain

- Decompresses the spinal nerves, facilitating normal nerve function and reducing nerve pain

- Improves circulation around the spine and to the arms, supporting better tissue health and repair

- Reduces stress on other spinal structures

- Increases the safety margin for everyday movements that distort the spine (fig.1-7)

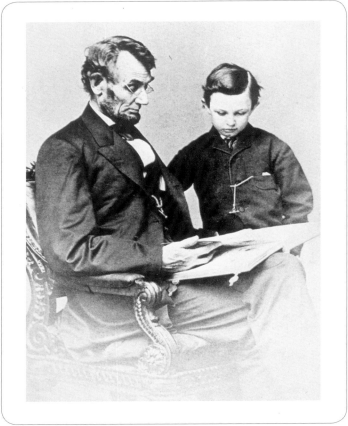

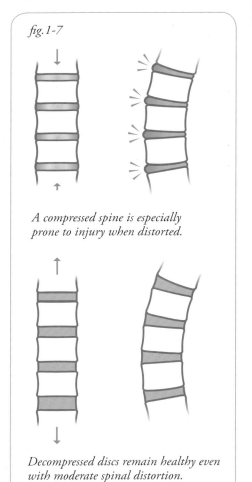

fig.1-7

A compressed spine is especially prone to injury when distorted.

Decompressed discs remain healthy even with moderate spinal distortion.

I am amazed at how much more comfortable I am in everyday life and while traveling.

Rebecca Barfknecht, Chief Technology Officer, Charles Schwab & Co., San Francisco, CA

For many years, I basically "put up with" an intermittent yet chronic lower back pain. Exercise helped offer temporary relief, but days of sitting in the office all day brought it right back. A colleague with much more serious back problems recommended I see Esther. Her praise of the benefits was encouraging, but I kept putting it off as something I could do by myself. I never thought of myself as having "bad posture." What I came to realize is that most people (in our society anyway) have some degree of bad posture. I felt the benefits from day one. I rarely have back pain now, and I feel more healthy and energetic overall. I am very pleased to testify to the positive effects of this work.

John Hamilton, Geologist (USGS) and musician, Menlo Park, CA

fig. 1-8

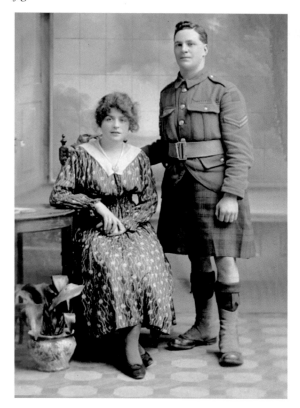

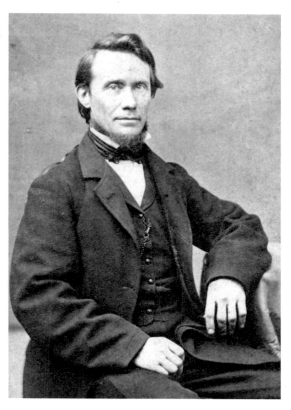

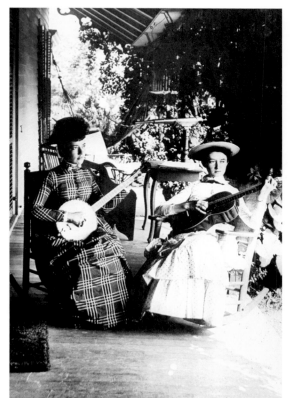

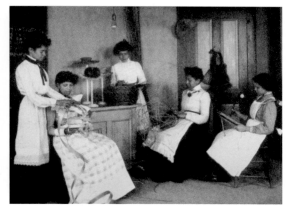

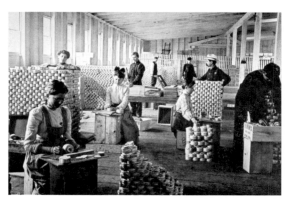

Examples of people from former times sitting with a healthy baseline length in their back muscles (USA)

EQUIPMENT

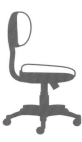

You will need a suitable chair, such as a secretarial chair or padded folding chair. The ideal is a chair with:

- *A firm seat*
- *A low, straight backrest that, if adjustable, can be locked into position*
- *An outcropping at the mid-back level to which you can "hitch" your spine*

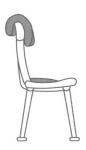

If your chair lacks an outcropping, you can fashion one from a folded towel or flannel sheet that you place just below your shoulder blades. The folded material:

- *Offers a place to hitch your mid-back*
- *Gives your buttocks space to settle behind you in the chair*
- *Provides enough clearance to let you perform a shoulder roll*

See page 228 for information on ordering a backrest I developed, which you can use on any chair.

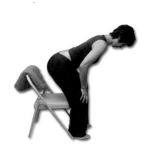
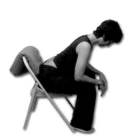

1 SIT DOWN, PLACING YOUR BUTTOCKS WELL BACK IN THE CHAIR

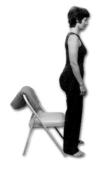

If the chair has a gap between the seat and the back, be careful not to place your buttocks too far back. If you do, your back will sway in later steps.

2 PLACE YOUR FEET ABOUT HIP-WIDTH APART AND RELAX YOUR LEGS

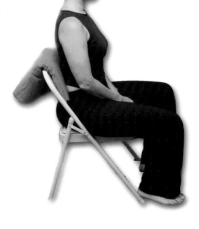

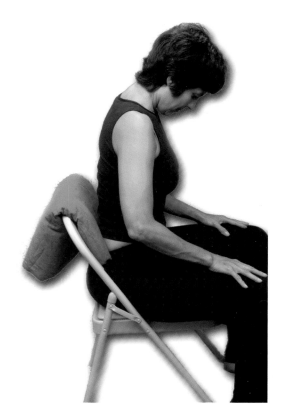

3 LENGTHEN YOUR SPINE

Bend at the waist and curve forward slightly to lengthen your low back. This eliminates any sway you may have, and prevents your introducing one in the next step.

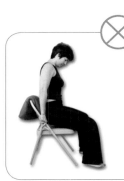

4 FURTHER LENGTHEN YOUR SPINE

Leave your buttocks anchored to the chair. With both hands, hold on to some part of the chair (armrests, backrest, or seat) and push with your arms. Relax the muscles of your torso, allowing the rib cage to separate as much as possible from the pelvis.

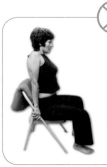

A common mistake is to arch backwards, which actually shortens the spine instead of lengthening it.

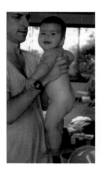

Another common mistake is to raise the buttocks out of the chair.

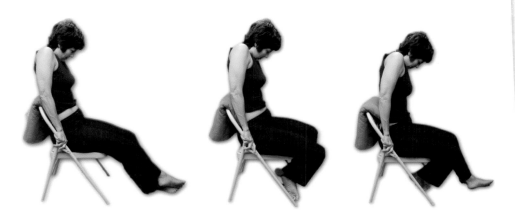

Be sure you are not engaging your leg muscles in this step. If you find they are tense, stretch your legs forward, fold them under your chair, or use any relaxed position.

ROTATING THE RIB CAGE FORWARD TO LENGTHEN THE LOW BACK

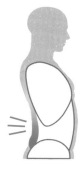
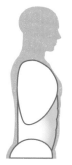

Compromised   *Ideal*

EXAMPLES OF STRETCHING THE SPINE IN EVERYDAY LIFE

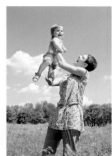

These photos show a maneuver familiar to us all: lifting a baby, helping to lengthen its spine.

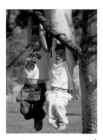
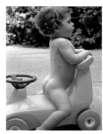

Many common childhood activities lengthen the spine.

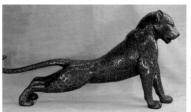

We often see animals stretching their spines.

© Donald Greig

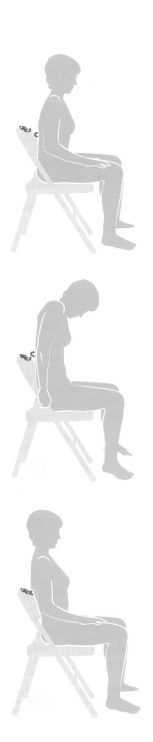

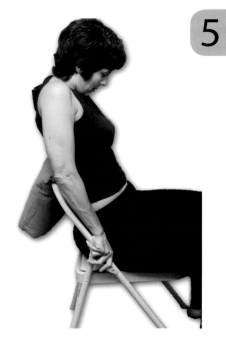

5 ATTACH YOUR MID-BACK TO THE BACKREST OR CUSHION

Keeping your arms engaged to maintain the extra length in your spine, "hitch" your back to the backrest of the chair. Think of pinning a point in your mid-back as high as possible on the backrest. For most people, this will be about an inch higher than normal.

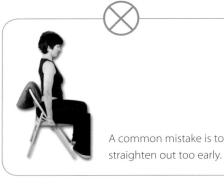

A common mistake is to straighten out too early.

6 RELEASE THE TENSION IN YOUR ARMS

Feel the chair take the weight as you release your arms.

It may help to imagine that you hang from the point of contact with the chair like a picture hangs from a picture hook.

7 STRAIGHTEN YOUR UPPER BACK

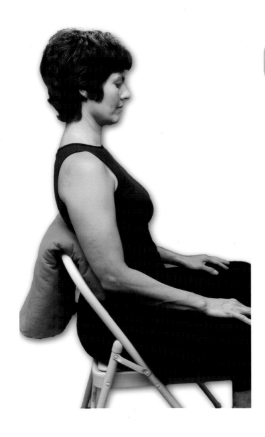

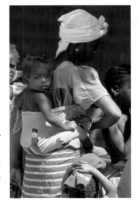

Mother carrying baby. Fabric stretches baby's back (Burkina Faso)

Now your lower back is in traction.   Be sure not to arch back over the chair nor to press so hard against the backrest as to cause discomfort.

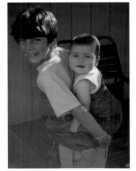

Girl using traditional African technique to carry baby (USA)

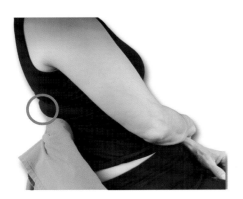

If your lower back feels stretched out, you are right on track even though it feels strange at first. If you are not sure that you have succeeded in stretching your lower back, place a hand on your back just above the point of contact with the chair. You should feel a roll of skin there. The chair stretches your skin and eases your vertebrae apart.

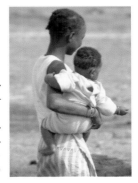

Teenager carrying baby on hip, stretching the baby's back with forearm (Burkina Faso)

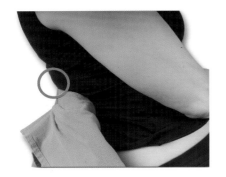

If you are uncomfortable, try backing off a little so as to lengthen in a more subtle manner. It is important that you lengthen, but not that you achieve an ideal length overnight. Proceed gently.

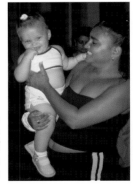

Woman facilitating baby's mild spinal stretch (Brazil)

MECHANISM OF A SHOULDER ROLL

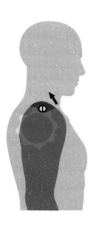

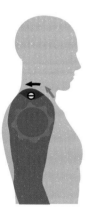

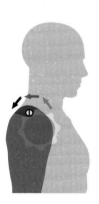

When doing a shoulder roll, imagine the shoulder's soft tissue ratcheting back one notch on a cogged wheel. Unless the pectoral muscles are very tight, the shoulders tend to remain in this position without any sustained muscular effort. (See Appendix 1 for exercises to help stretch tight pectoral muscles.)

8 PERFORM A SHOULDER ROLL WITH EACH SHOULDER

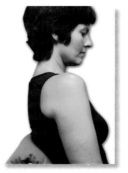

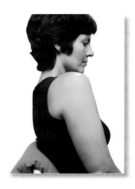

Hunch one shoulder forward, causing it to round.

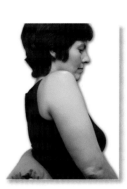

Lift the shoulder toward your ears.

As with all the movements you learn in this book, the shoulder roll may feel exaggerated and awkward at first, something you wouldn't be comfortable doing in public. With practice and time, the movement becomes subtle, and you can easily incorporate it into seating yourself at a company meeting, in a restaurant, or on your sofa.

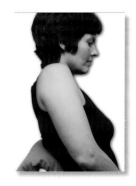

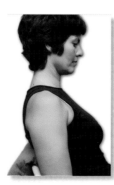

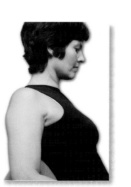

Gently slide the shoulder blade down along your spine.

Roll the shoulder back as far as you comfortably can.

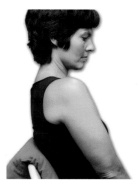 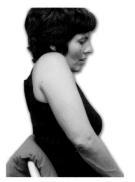 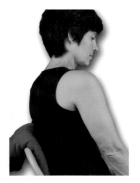

Common mistakes are to over-exaggerate the movement, do it too abruptly, or move the arm more than the shoulder blade.

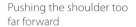

Pushing the shoulder too far forward

Raising the shoulder too high

Moving the arm excessively

After performing a shoulder roll, you may notice that your reach is shorter. This is because your arms now originate further back than before. This is a healthy home base position that you don't want to compromise during normal activities. The solution is to adjust your distance from your task. For example, when working at a computer, you may need to move the keyboard closer. When driving a car, you may need to move your car seat closer to the steering wheel (but keep a safe distance from the airbag).

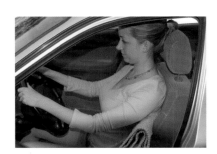

Driving with shoulders well-positioned

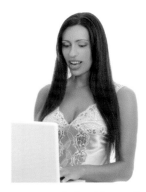

Typing with shoulders well-positioned

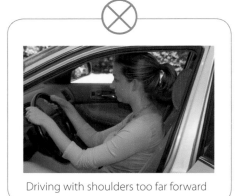

Driving with shoulders too far forward

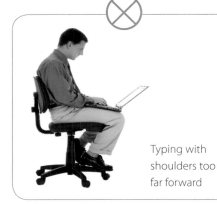

Typing with shoulders too far forward

EXAMPLES OF GOOD SHOULDER ALIGNMENT

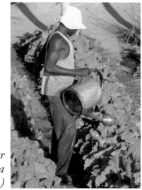

Farmer (Burkina Faso)

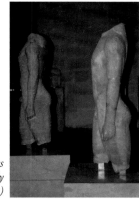

Statues (early Greece)

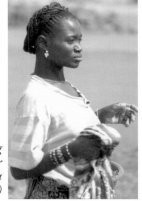

Young mother (Burkina Faso)

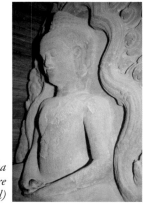

Buddha figure (Thailand)

43

HEALTHY NECK POSTURE FROM AROUND THE WORLD

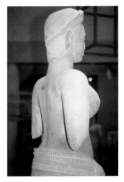

Boddhisattva figure (Cambodia)

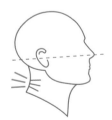

Young mother (Burkina Faso)

ROTATING THE HEAD FORWARD TO LENGTHEN THE NECK

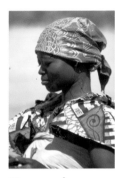

Compromised

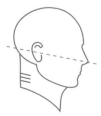

Ideal

9 LENGTHEN THE BACK OF YOUR NECK

Though you have lengthened your back, your neck may still be compressed. There are many ways to lengthen the neck. If your neck is injury-prone, choose Option A or a very gentle version of Option B. If you are looking to make fast progress, use Option E occasionally. Otherwise, choose according to what is comfortable for you. The goal is a neutral neck position with the jaw gliding back and up and the chin angled down.

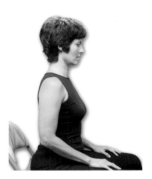

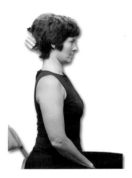

Option A. Imagine a helium balloon inside your head. Consciously release any tension in your neck muscles that works against the balloon's upward thrust.

Option B. Grab a clump of hair at the base of your skull and gently pull it back and up.

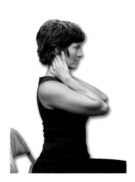

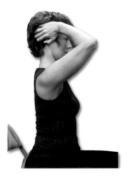

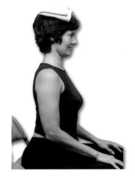

Option C. Position your fingertips in the two side indentations at the base of your skull (the *occipital grooves*) and move your skull up and away from your body.

Option D. Grasp the base of your skull with both hands and gently pull upward while lowering your shoulders.

Option E. Place (or imagine) a light object on the crown of your head. Push up against it.

If there is some rigidity in your neck, your head and neck may still crane forward. See the Appendix 1 for exercises to help stretch rigid neck muscles.

⊗

Try to avoid these common mistakes:

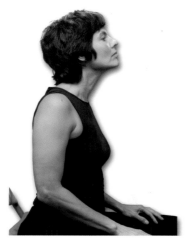

Do not lengthen the front of your neck instead of the back.

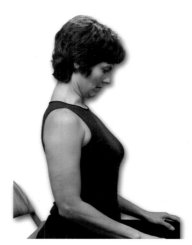

Do not tuck your chin into your neck as you lengthen the back of your neck.

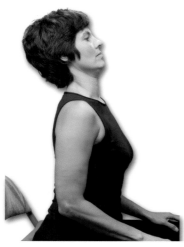

Do not tilt your head back in an attempt to lengthen the neck.

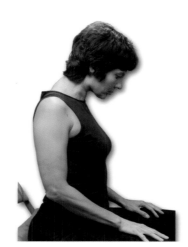

Do not jut your head forward and tilt your chin down as you lengthen the back of your neck.

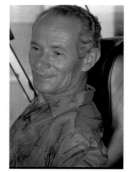

Man on bus (Brazil)

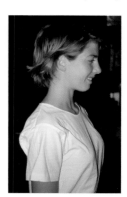

College student (USA)

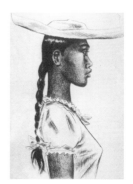

Drawing of girl (Tahiti)

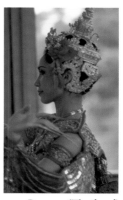

Dancer (Thailand)

HEALTHY FOOT SHAPE AROUND THE WORLD

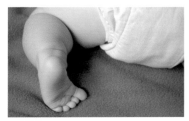

Six-month-old infant with pronounced kidney-bean shaped foot (USA)

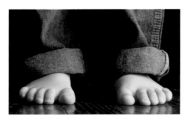

Young child showing healthy toe spacing (USA)

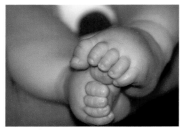

Baby with pronounced transverse arches in the feet (USA)

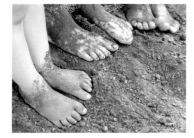

Children with sturdy feet from walking on natural surfaces (India)

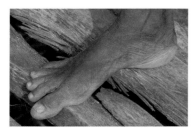

Laborer with muscular, healthy feet (India)

10 WHILE CONTINUING TO STRETCHSIT, FIX THE TOES AND BALL OF ONE FOOT ON THE FLOOR WHILE LIFTING THE HEEL

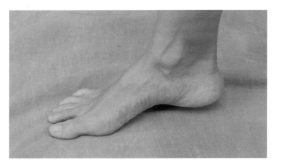

Lift foot just high enough so that the heel clears the floor.

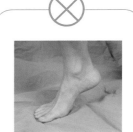

A common mistake is to lift the heel too high, tensing the foot muscles and making the next step difficult.

11 TWIST AND PIVOT THE HEEL INWARD BEFORE PLANTING IT FIRMLY ON THE FLOOR

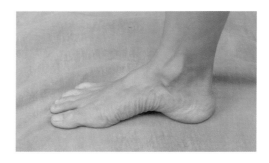

Your goal is to create a "kidney-bean" shape with your foot.

12 REPEAT THIS ACTION WITH THE OTHER FOOT

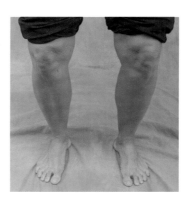

Notice that your knees point in the same direction as your toes.

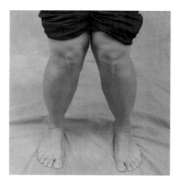

A common mistake is to pronate the feet and turn the knees in, which causes misalignment in the entire leg, pelvis, and spine.

13 RELAX YOUR WHOLE BODY

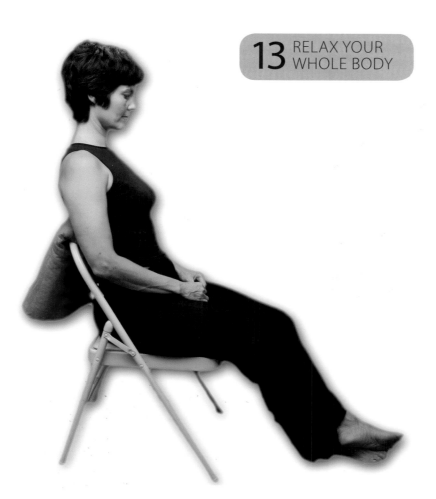

Let the chair do all the work. Try to locate any tension in your body and release it. Reposition your legs as you wish.

If you find that you settle back to your habitual position after a while, you will need to reset your position periodically. Simply repeat the steps of this lesson.

SITTING WITH AN ELONGATED SPINE

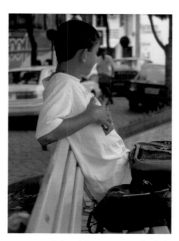

School boy sitting slightly reclined while lengthening his back (Brazil)

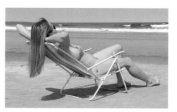

Woman reclining on a beach chair while elongating her neck (USA)

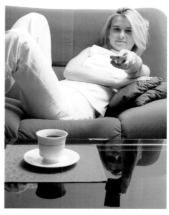

Woman propped on sofa with cushions supporting her spine (USA)

Stretchsitting does not oblige you to sit bolt upright. As long as your spine is elongated and its natural curves respected, you will be comfortable and protected in a variety of positions ranging from upright to reclining.

INDICATIONS OF IMPROVEMENT

With practice, you will learn how to stretchsit quickly and easily. Usually this sitting position, though unfamiliar at first, becomes very comfortable. It allows you to sit for extended periods without squirming. Eventually, the resting length of your back will change, your height will be measurably taller, and you will be more comfortable even when you are not in traction.

Over time, your lengthened back muscles will contribute to improved circulation (which in turn hastens healing of damage), and will help to decompress discs and nerves - all with the result of increased comfort and function. Because most nerves in the body originate in the spinal column, normalizing this area will improve your general well-being.

You may also notice gradual changes in your breathing pattern. To track this, pay attention to which parts of your body move during a breath cycle. Place one hand on your chest and one hand on your abdomen to check the relative movement in these two areas (fig.1-9). When you have lengthened your spine and opened your shoulders, you will probably notice more movement in your chest and less in your abdomen. Though abdominal breathing is natural during exertion, chest breathing during rest expands lung capacity and supports the normal architecture of the rib cage.

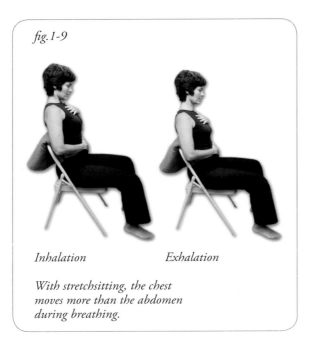

fig.1-9

Inhalation   *Exhalation*

With stretchsitting, the chest moves more than the abdomen during breathing.

TROUBLESHOOTING

FEELING OVERLY STRETCHED

If you feel as though you are on a rack, you may have stretched yourself too severely. Ease the stretch by moving slightly away from the backrest and letting your upper back slide down the backrest just a little (fig.1-10).

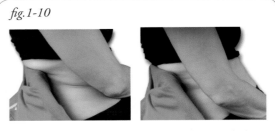

fig.1-10

If a strong stretch (with a pronounced roll of flesh) feels uncomfortable, back off a little.

UNABLE TO STRETCH THE SPINE

If after following the directions in this chapter you don't feel a stretch in your spine, check for a telltale roll of flesh above the point of contact with the chair. If you find it, you are actually stretchsitting but just not feeling it yet. In time, you will probably begin to feel the stretch.

If your arms are weak or injured, you may not be able to use them effectively to lengthen your torso. Reach your hands around to your mid-back, and stretch the skin on your back upwards before hitching yourself to the backrest (fig.1-11). Alternatively, if your chair is stable, you can use your legs to help push your back higher up against the backrest (fig.1-12).

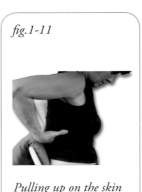

fig.1-11

Pulling up on the skin of the back is another effective way to lengthen the back for stretchsitting.

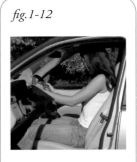

fig.1-12

With a stable chair or car seat, pushing with the legs can help to position you for stretchsitting.

If you are still unable to lengthen your spine, you may be having difficulty relaxing your abdominal and back muscles enough to allow any separation between your upper body and your lower body. Try consciously to relax the muscles in your torso as you stretch your back (except those you need to curve forward slightly) and proceed very slowly.

If your muscles feel very tight, you may benefit from some supplemental bodywork. Consider yoga, massage, acupuncture, and stretching exercises.

DISCOMFORT AT POINT OF CONTACT

If the place where your back contacts the chair feels sore, you may have some inflammation there. Arrange the support cushion a little higher or lower to avoid this spot. If you still have trouble, you may want to skip to the next lesson until you can perform this exercise comfortably. Consider massage or acupuncture to help resolve the inflammation.

INADEQUATE CHAIR

Some chairs are difficult to modify. Try different combinations of chairs and back supports. Don't settle for anything less than an extremely comfortable sitting position. One way to modify almost any chair is with the backrest I have designed for stretchsitting (fig.1-13).

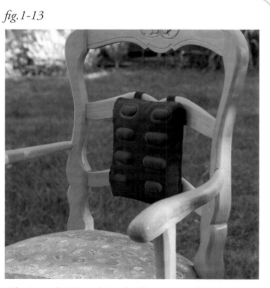

fig.1-13

The Stretchsit™ cushion facilitates stretchsitting in almost any chair. To order, see www.egwellness.com

FURTHER INFORMATION

SHOULDER REPOSITIONING

Most people who recognize they have poor posture know that their shoulders hunch forward. Unfortunately, the ways they know to fix the problem are either ineffective or harmful.

A common approach to correcting hunched shoulders is to pull them directly back (fig.1-14). People usually hold this position about 10 seconds before they again slouch their shoulders – until the next time they become aware they are hunching. The movement of pulling the shoulders back involves contracting the *rhomboid* muscles, which is a good exercise but a bad way to correct one's posture. It is just as well that people don't hold this position for long: If they did, they would suffer inflammation from overuse of the rhomboids.

Another common, and worse, compensation for hunched shoulders is to sway the low back (fig.1-15). This approach creates two problems in place of one. The original hunching remains unresolved, and the low back is compromised as well. Sometimes this combination of excessive curvatures is mistakenly perceived as good posture, because the upper body appears upright.

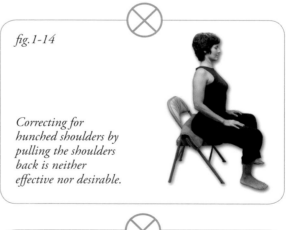

fig.1-14

Correcting for hunched shoulders by pulling the shoulders back is neither effective nor desirable.

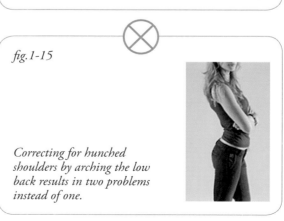

fig.1-15

Correcting for hunched shoulders by arching the low back results in two problems instead of one.

Performing careful shoulder rolls is the best way to remedy hunching. Shoulder rolls influence the architecture of the area just beneath the pectoral muscles. This area, called the *brachial plexus*, is a major thoroughfare for nerves and blood vessels supplying the arms. Hunching the shoulders compromises the architecture of this area, affecting blood supply to and from the arms, and nerve function in the arms. Symptoms range from cold hands and dry skin to arm pain and dysfunction.

Shoulder rolls are relatively easy to learn and perform. If you have extremely tight pectoral muscles, you should proceed gently with shoulder rolls. Otherwise, your overstretched muscles may press down and impinge on underlying blood vessels and nerves. For exercises to help you progress faster towards well-aligned shoulders, see Appendix 1.

COMMENTS ON LUMBAR CUSHIONS

A common solution for an uncomfortable chair or seat is a lumbar support cushion that supports and even exaggerates lumbar curvature (fig.1-16a). The design of these cushions is based on misguided notions about ideal spinal curvature. Even when placed above the lumbar spine, most lumbar cushions do not work for stretchsitting, as they don't have the appropriate firmness or texture for "hitching" the spine.

I designed my Stretchsit™ cushion for effective hitching, and for easy attachment to most seats at the appropriate height (fig.1-16b). The backrest helps to lengthen the lumbar spine, making sitting a comfortable and therapeutic position.

SITTING IN A CAR

This lesson would be incomplete without describing how to sit in a car. Because so many of us sit for hours every week in our cars, it is essential to spend those hours sitting well. You may remember a time when riding in a car was so comfortable that you called it "joy riding." With age, too many of us find that even a short road trip causes discomfort or pain. When you succeed in positioning yourself well, you will again find that driving is a pleasure, and you will no longer arrive at your destination feeling pain or stiffness.

Stretchsitting is especially important when driving. Using the instructions in this section will enable you to elongate your spine in your car. The extra space you gain between the vertebrae acts as a buffer against the motions of the car. It also counteracts the extra compression that can result from muscle tension when driving in stressful conditions.

Most car seats are poorly designed, including those with numerous adjustments. This is because they are made to reflect the average posture of the people using them. Unfortunately, they also perpetuate this average posture. The seats are too concave both vertically and horizontally. They push the driver's shoulders forward, causing the back to hunch (fig.1-17). They offer no place to hitch the thoracic spine and no possibility of doing a shoulder roll. However, you can remedy these problems by placing a support so that it rests at the level of the mid-back, just below the shoulder blades.

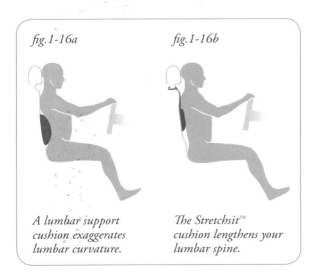

fig.1-16a *fig.1-16b*

A lumbar support cushion exaggerates lumbar curvature.

The Stretchsit™ cushion lengthens your lumbar spine.

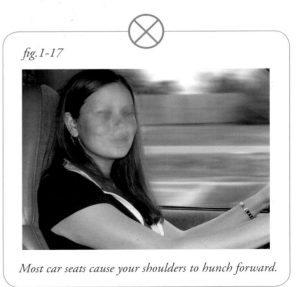

fig.1-17

Most car seats cause your shoulders to hunch forward.

FASHIONING A BACKREST

The trick is to fold a piece of fabric into the appropriate shape for your back (fig.1-18a). The exact dimensions will depend on the contours of your car seat. The more curved your car seat, the thicker the cushion should be. In cars with slippery leather seats, position folded material vertically, jamming one end between the headrest and the back of the seat (fig.1-18b). The rest of the material should drape down the seat to the level of the mid back in a strip that fits between the shoulder blades. Be sure that your head still reaches the headrest. Or use my Stretchsit℠ cushion, which works by fastening around the headrest in all car seats (fig.1-18c).

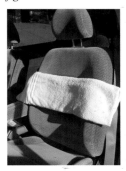

fig.1-18a

Folded fabric can modify a car seat for healthy posture.

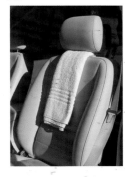

fig.1-18b

Some ingenuity is needed to modify leather seats for healthy posture.

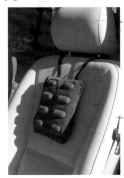

fig.1-18c

The Stretchsit™ cushion has a strap that attaches around the headrest.

Once you have modified your car seat, the steps are similar to those for stretchsitting in a chair with a backrest:

1. Shift your buttocks back into the seat relative to your upper body.

2. Lengthen your back against the backrest and place your back in traction. Rather than using just your arms to hoist your torso onto the outcropping, you may find it helpful to push with your legs (fig.1-12). This works in a car because the seat is fixed and stable.

3. Perform a shoulder roll to move your shoulders back and down. Because of the backrest, your shoulders should not be impeded by the poor contours of the seat.

4. Check and adjust your distance to the steering wheel. You should be close enough to comfortably reach the wheel without rounding your shoulders. Note: Be sure to follow the manufacturer's guidelines for maintaining a safe distance from the air bags.

5. Try to lengthen your neck. Just as you can place your torso in traction against the cushion, you may be able to place your neck in traction against the headrest (fig.1-19).

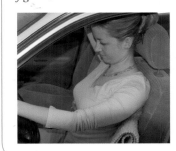

fig.1-19

Lengthen your neck against the headrest to get gentle traction in your neck.

CHECKING YOUR POSITION

You can use the position of your rearview mirror to set a standard for your seated height. Seat yourself as directed in these instructions and then adjust the rearview mirror to give you good rear vision. Now, whenever you drive, be sure you sit so that you can use the mirror in its established position. Don't adjust the mirror; adjust how you sit!

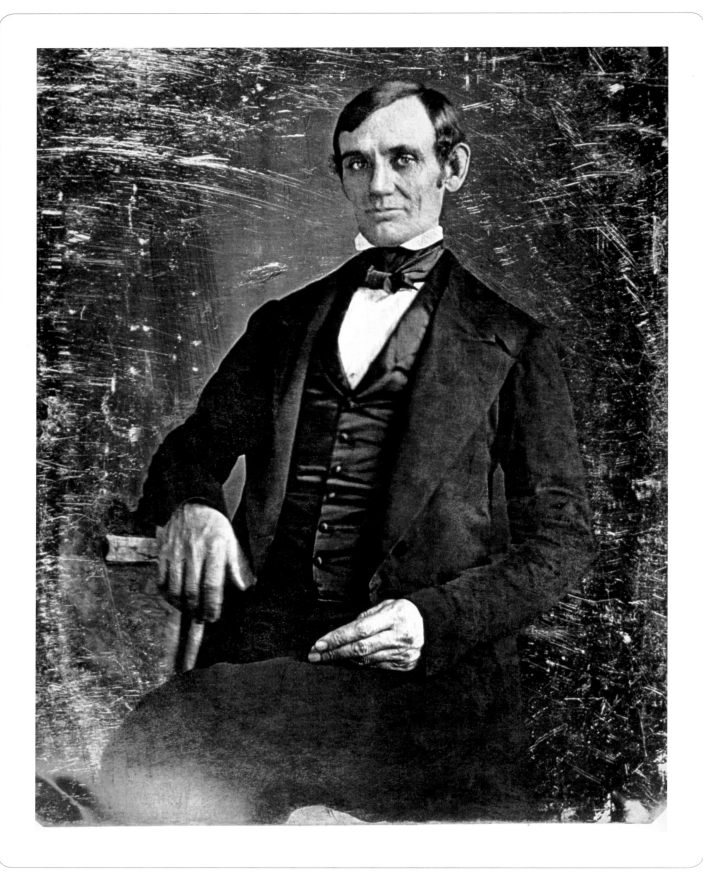

RECAP

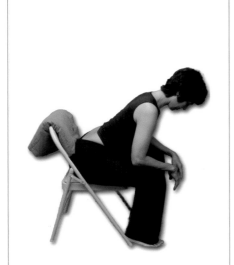

a. Sit on chair, moving buttocks well back in chair

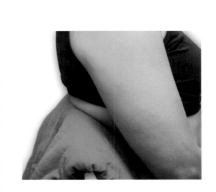

b. Lengthen spine

c. Attach mid-back to chair

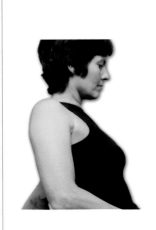

d. Perform shoulder rolls

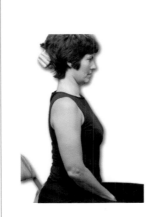

e. Lengthen back of neck

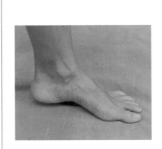

f. Align feet in kidney bean shape

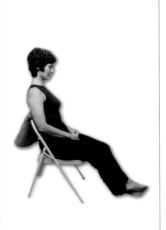

g. Relax entire body

2

STRETCHLYING ON YOUR BACK

Lying with a lengthened back

My youngest daughter sleeps peacefully as a baby. Notice the dome-like contour of her chest, her upper back and neck in a straight line, her sacrum (the lowest part of her back) angled posteriorly leaving a gap between it and the bed, and her head turned on the axis of the spine.

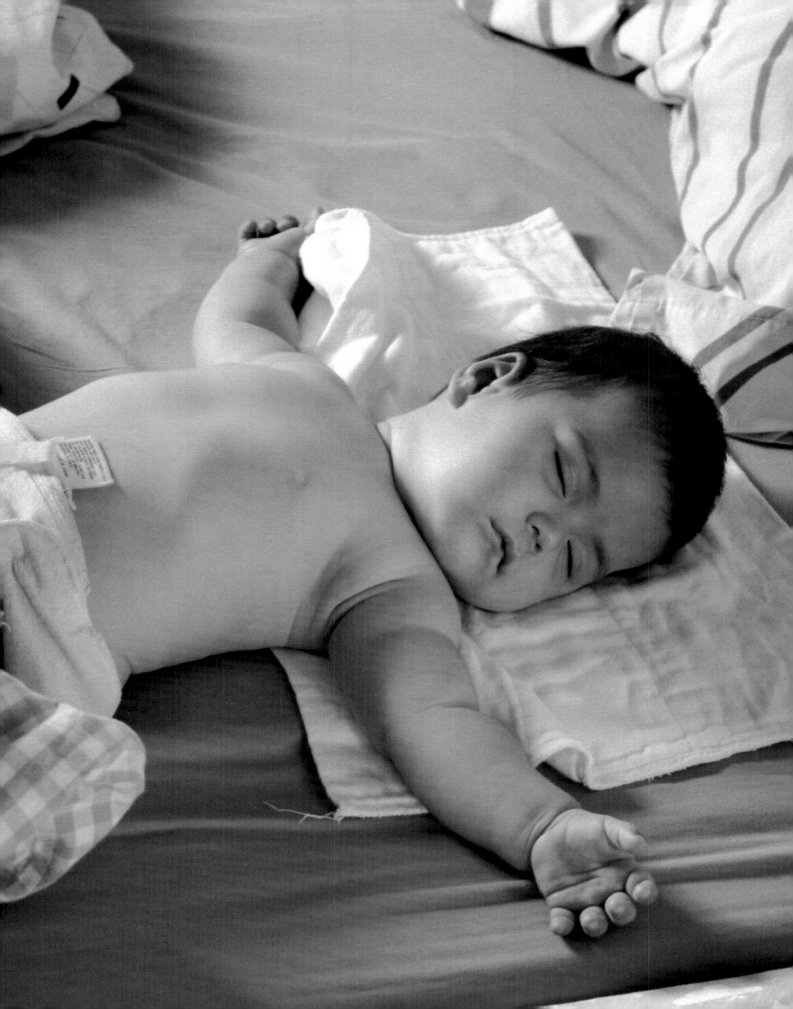

In this lesson you will learn the technique of stretchlying to elongate your spine when you lie down (fig.2-1). With this and the sitting position that you learned in the first lesson, you will gain therapeutic benefit for many hours each day – far more than that provided in any normal stretching regimen. Not only will you benefit from hours of therapeutic traction for your back, but you will also enjoy improved sleep.

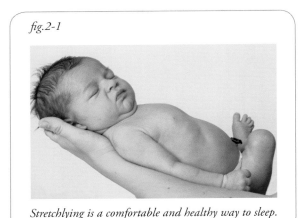

fig.2-1

Stretchlying is a comfortable and healthy way to sleep.

A good night's sleep is nature's way of restoring and resetting the body, yet many people experience the night hours as a time of discomfort, restlessness, and even pain. Most of us understand the connection between emotions and sleep; fewer people understand the role of our sleep position.

A poor sleep position threatens various body structures, which in turn signal the brain to change position. Tossing and turning is an attempt to find a healthy position in which your muscles can relax. If you don't succeed, and remain in an unhealthy position, you may well wake up with aches and pains because your muscles did not relax during the night (fig.2-2).

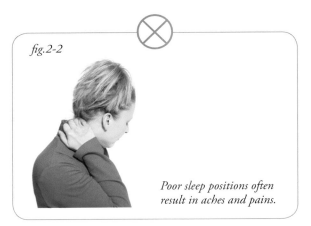

fig.2-2

Poor sleep positions often result in aches and pains.

If you start the night with your body in a relaxed, neutral position, you won't have to toss and turn to find one. You may be surprised by how long you remain in one position, and by how refreshed and comfortable you feel upon waking. Indeed, many people report waking in the same position after a whole night's sleep once they have learned stretchlying.

When you have mastered the technique, it will only require a few seconds each night to get into an optimal position and enjoy improved sleep.

If you do not normally sleep on your back, you may question the value of this lesson, but I encourage you to learn stretchlying for several reasons:

- You may surprise yourself by falling asleep in the stretchlying position.
- Even if you do not fall asleep, you will benefit from starting out the night with lengthened back muscles. They will retain some of the length even after you move out of this position.
- It is useful to cultivate more than one comfortable and healthy sleeping position to accommodate special circumstances, such as an injury.
- Many common exercises are performed lying on your back; stretchlying makes the exercises safer.
- Massage and other bodywork techniques usually require lying on the back. Again, stretchlying makes bodywork safer, more comfortable, and more effective.

When you first try a new sleep position, it may feel contrived, cumbersome, and not conducive to sleep. It takes some discipline to start the night in a strange position, even when it feels very comfortable. If you use this discipline for three or four nights, the strangeness will wear off and be replaced by positive feelings.

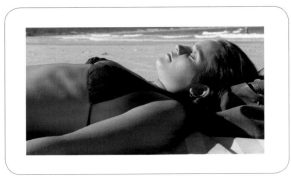

BENEFITS

- Improves quality of sleep

- Decompresses spinal discs

- Decompresses spinal nerves

- Improves circulation around the spine

- Resets the resting length of back muscles

- Improves breathing pattern

I noticed that I began to sleep more soundly, without tossing and turning throughout the night, and when I woke up in the morning I didn't feel the need to stretch in order to move, as I had in the past. My circulation is much better now and I haven't had a physical injury in ages. Everybody comments on "What good posture I have!!"

Merrill Page, Stanford student, Stanford, CA

The pain was so severe that my entire body was tense trying to fight it. There was no relief at night. No position would alleviate the throbbing. I would wake up as tense and weary as when I went to bed. People noticed the limp and the dragging of my left leg. Walking the dog was torture. Trying to mask the pain became impossible. Thoughts of surgery filled me with dread.

One of my friends suggested Esther Gokhale, who had helped her boss resolve recurring pain. I shall admit that I was skeptical. After my first session I walked out feeling better, but I believed that the relief would be short lived. That whole week was a week with minimal pain. I am still going to Esther. I have had a total of six visits. Learning is challenging. I have had no pain for four weeks. The work is not always easy, but the payoff is probably as close to a miracle as I'll ever get.

Smokey Chapman,
Palo Alto, CA

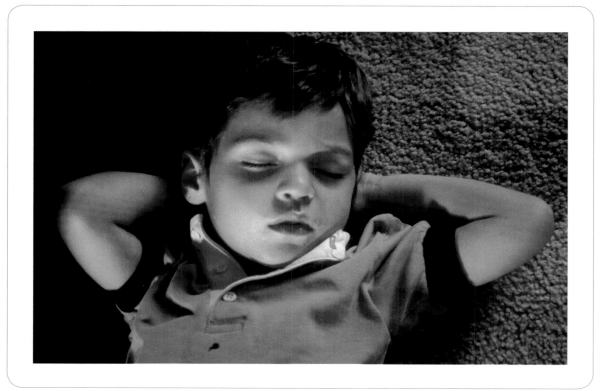

EQUIPMENT

You will need the following:
- *Two pillows, one for under your head and one for under your knees (See Further Information on page 65 for guidance on pillow thickness.)*
- *A bed*

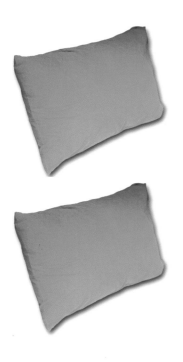

1 SIT WITH YOUR KNEES BENT AND YOUR FEET FLAT ON THE BED

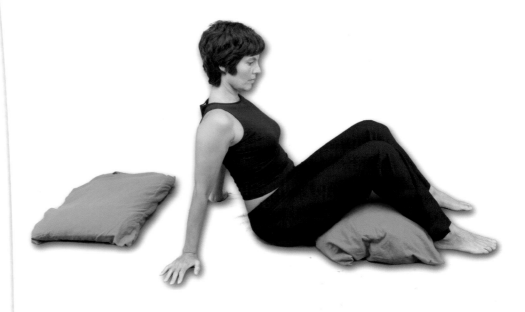

Your legs should be over (not resting on) a pillow.

2 USING YOUR ELBOWS, LOWER YOUR UPPER BODY TO ABOUT A 30° ANGLE

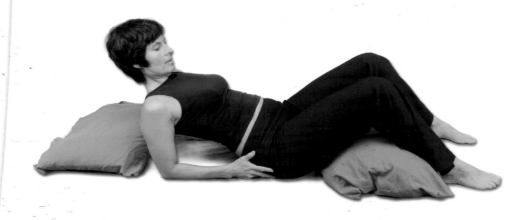

Bend your arms so your forearms are resting on the bed and your elbows form a 90° angle with the bed.

3 SLOWLY LOWER YOUR BACK ONTO THE BED WHILE LENGTHENING YOUR SPINE

IDEAL AND COMPROMISED WAYS TO LIE ON YOUR BACK

Press your elbows into the bed and down toward your feet to help elongate your spine. Focus on lowering your back onto the bed vertebra by vertebra, positioning each vertebra as far from the previous one as possible. When your elbows no longer give leverage, lie down the rest of the way, placing your head and upper shoulders on a pillow.

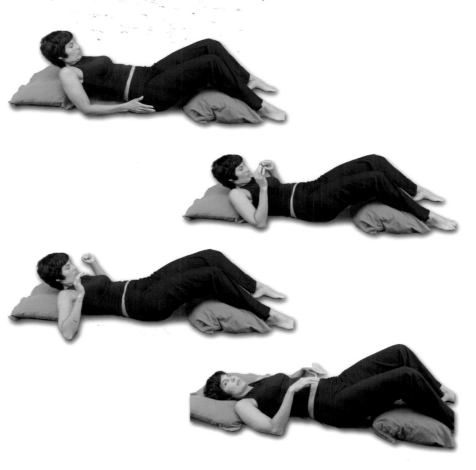

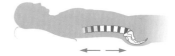

Lying stretched

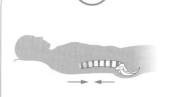

Lying compressed

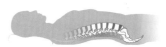

Lying swayed

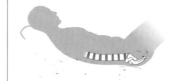

Lying rounded

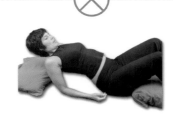

A common mistake is to arch the back as you attempt to lengthen it. In fact, arching shortens the back. Concentrate on positioning each vertebra as far from the previous one as possible.

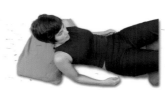

A nearly universal tendency is to over-tuck the pelvis. With the discs decompressed by stretchlying, this will likely do no harm. However, if you feel any discomfort, use the maneuver in Step 10.

IDEAL AND COMPROMISED SHOULDER AND NECK POSITIONS

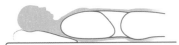

A pillow under the shoulders flattens the low back.

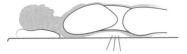

No pillow under shoulders can result in a swayed low back.

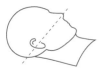

Elongated neck

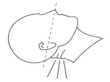

Compressed neck

EXAMPLES OF HEALTHY NECK POSITION

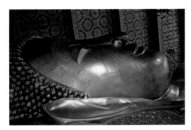

Reclining Buddha (Thailand)

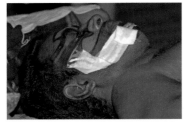

Kathakali dancer having make-up applied (India)

60

4 CHECK THE POSITION OF YOUR PILLOW

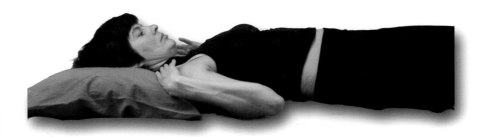

Your shoulders, neck, and head should be slightly raised on the edge of the pillow. You may have to adjust the position of the pillow if, after elongating your spine, you are too high or low on the pillow.

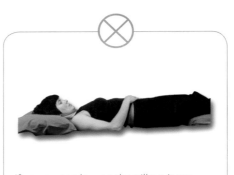

If you are too low on the pillow, it can cause your neck to curve forward.

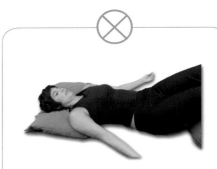

If you are too high on the pillow, it can cause your neck to sway.

5 GENTLY ELONGATE YOUR NECK

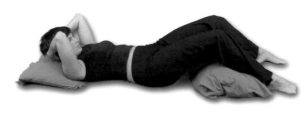

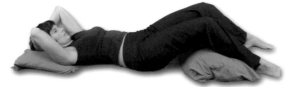

Lift your head from the pillow. Use your hands to guide the back of head away from your torso as you lay your head back down on the pillow. It is important to do this gently.

6 SLIDE YOUR SHOULDERS DOWN ALONG YOUR SPINE

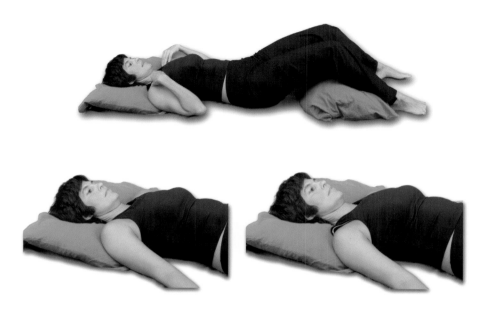

Earlier, you used your elbows to position your back, so now your shoulders may be hiked up towards your ears. Because you cannot complete a full shoulder roll with the cushion behind your shoulders, simply slide your shoulders down, and widen across your chest.

7 POSITION YOUR ARMS COMFORTABLY AT YOUR SIDES

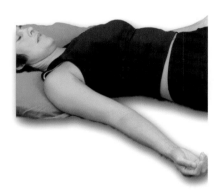
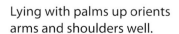
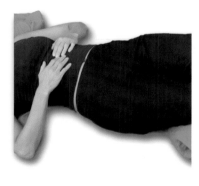

Lying with palms up orients arms and shoulders well.

Some people find it comfortable to bend their arms softly at the elbow, resting their hands on their abdomen. Others prefer to rest their arms under or above the head.

HEALTHY ARM POSITIONS

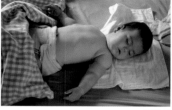

(USA)

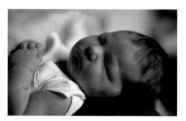

(USA)

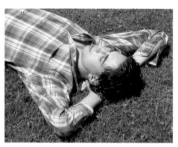

(USA)

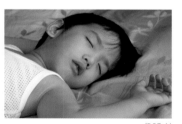

(USA)

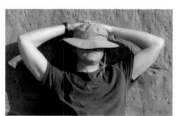

(USA)

COMPENSATING FOR TIGHT PSOAS MUSCLES

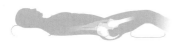

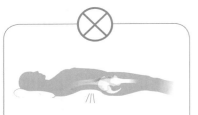

Placing a pillow under the knees compensates for tight psoas muscles, which originate at the front of the lumbar spine and end at the top of the femurs.

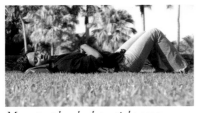

Lying with outstretched legs can cause a sway if the psoas muscles are tight.

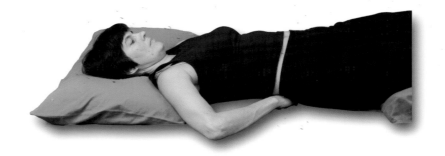

Many people who have tight psoas muscles instinctively bend their knees to facilitate a better alignment in the low back (USA).

For an exercise to stretch the psoas muscles, see Appendix 1.

8 STRAIGHTEN AND RELAX YOUR LEGS ONTO THE PILLOW

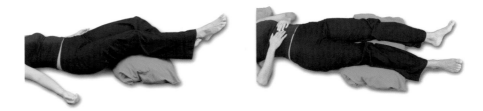

Gently rotate your legs and knees outward from the hip joint. The pillow beneath your knees supports them in a slightly bent position, relieving stress on your low back.

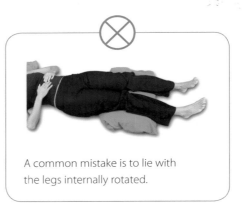

A common mistake is to lie with the legs internally rotated.

9 CHECK FOR A GAP BETWEEN YOUR LOW BACK AND THE BED

Sense whether your low back is in contact with the bed, or whether you can slide the fingers of one hand into a natural gap between your back and the bed. If there is no gap, your spine is not in a neutral position. Chances are you are in a strong tuck, which you will release in the next step.

10 IF YOUR PELVIS IS TUCKED, REPEAT THE STEPS IN THIS LESSON, STEADYING YOUR PELVIS WITH YOUR HANDS IN STEP 3

HEALTHY RECLINING POSITIONS

When lengthening your spine in Step 3, it is easy to unwittingly tuck your pelvis. The most effective way for your hands to steady your pelvis is with the fingers facing toward your feet and the thumb hooked behind the rim of your pelvis (the iliac crests).

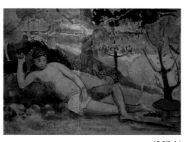

(USA)

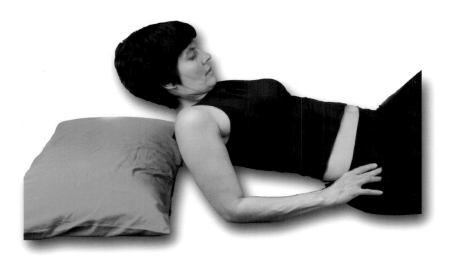

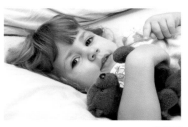

(USA)

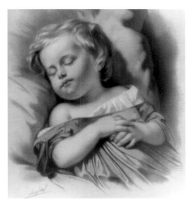

11 RELAX YOUR WHOLE BODY

Try to locate any tension in your body and release it. Lie in this position for two or three minutes, letting your muscles completely relax. If you are not already asleep and wish to stretch your spine even further, repeat steps 2-8.

(USA)

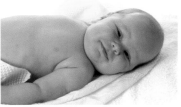

(USA)

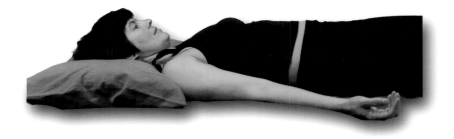

INDICATIONS OF IMPROVEMENT

When you spend an appreciable amount of time stretchlying, you will notice the same improvements as with stretchsitting: the resting length of your back will change, your height will be measurably taller, and you will be more comfortable even when not in traction. You will toss and turn less and experience better sleep.

Over time, your lengthened back muscles will contribute to improved circulation (which hastens healing of damage), and will help to decompress discs and nerves. Normalizing this area should improve your general well-being.

As with stretchsitting, you will also notice changes in your breathing pattern. To track this, pay attention to which parts of your body move as you breathe (fig.2-3). Place one hand on your chest and one hand on your abdomen to check their relative movement. You should notice more movement in your chest and less in your abdomen, because your stretched abdominal muscles now offer some resistance to belly breathing. Meanwhile, the improved alignment of the head, neck and upper torso facilitate easier movement in your chest. Over time, this increase in chest breathing will expand your lung capacity and support healthy architecture in your rib cage.

fig.2-3

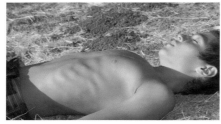

Inhalation

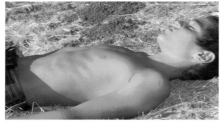

Exhalation

A healthy baseline breathing pattern expands the chest more than the abdomen.

TROUBLESHOOTING

FEELING PAIN OR DISCOMFORT IN THE LOW BACK

- You may have very tight psoas muscles causing your back to sway. Place more pillows under your knees to reduce the sway (fig.2-4).

fig.2-4

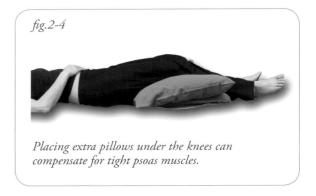

Placing extra pillows under the knees can compensate for tight psoas muscles.

- You may have over-tucked your pelvis as you lowered each vertebra onto the bed. If this has occurred, repeat Steps 1-8, this time placing your hands firmly on your pelvic rim to hold it stable (see Step10).

FEELING PAIN OR DISCOMFORT IN THE NECK

- You may have excessive neck curvature. Adjust the pillow to a height that is appropriate to the curvature in your neck and upper thoracic spine. You may even have to bunch the pillow up a little to form a "cervical roll," though make sure you are not encouraging your neck to curve more than it does already (fig.2-5). You are aiming for comfortable support and the elimination of tension. This may require experimentation with pillows of different firmness and thickness.

fig.2-5

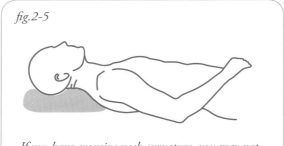

If you have excessive neck curvature, you may not be able to lengthen your neck a great deal. Support what curvature you have, and slowly work in the direction of lengthening the back of your neck.

- You may have overstretched your neck. If you feel uncomfortable, ease up a bit until you feel comfortable. Overstretching the neck muscles, especially if done abruptly, can trigger muscle spasms.

FEELING DISCOMFORT AT A POINT OF CONTACT WITH THE BED

You may have local inflammation that is causing discomfort. Sleep on your side for now (as described in Lesson 4, "Stretchlying on Your Side") and return to this technique later.

SNORING

Though good alignment can help reduce snoring even when you lie on your back, your problem may be too severe to overcome in this way. Sleep on your side rather than on your back to get a good night's sleep. If you suspect sleep apnea, consult a sleep expert.

FEELINGS OF EXPOSURE

You may feel exposed and vulnerable stretchlying on your back. Focus on the comfortable feeling in your body and you will likely soon get used to the new position.

FURTHER INFORMATION

BEDS

People often ask me for recommendations on beds. After learning to stretchlie, you will find that you tolerate a greater variety of sleep surfaces. For example, a night spent on a bed with a slight sag or on a hard surface will not cause damage or trigger protective tightening in the spinal muscles (fig.2-6). In stretchlying your discs are decompressed so they can tolerate distortions in the shape of the spine much better than compressed discs can.

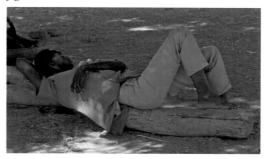

fig.2-6

If you have a decompressed spine, you will tolerate a wide range of mattress firmness. The "bed" in this photograph is extra-extra-firm, but is not causing the sleeper any problems (Burkina Faso).

An ideal bed is neither too firm nor too soft. It gives a little to accommodate the uneven contours of your body (especially important for wide-hipped, narrow-waisted women who sleep on their side), but does not let your heavier parts sink too deeply into the bed. The bed should not let your trunk sink too much relative to your arms, or your hips sink too much relative to your trunk. I recommend a high-quality, firm mattress with a high spring count.

PILLOWS

The right pillow for you depends on how much rigidity and curvature you have in your neck (*cervical*) and upper *thoracic* spine. A good pillow reflects your current baseline posture but encourages your neck to move in the direction of the ideal, albeit gradually (fig.2-7). It does not perpetuate or, worse, exaggerate unhealthy curvature (fig.2-8, fig.2-9). A good pillow has enough substance to hold a baseline shape, yet enough softness to be caressing and conducive to relaxation and sleep. One solution is to use two pillows - the lower one filled with a firm substance (like buckwheat hulls or kapok) and the upper one with a soft filling (like goosedown or synthetic fill).

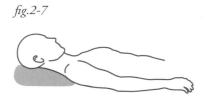
fig.2-7

A pillow placed under your head and slightly under your shoulders can serve to elongate your neck and low back.

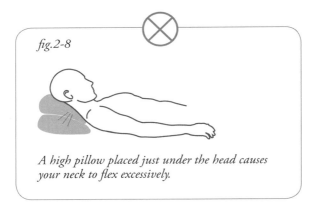
fig.2-8

A high pillow placed just under the head causes your neck to flex excessively.

CERVICAL PILLOWS / ROLLS

Cervical pillows and rolls, like lumbar cushions, are based on misguided notions about what constitutes normal and desirable curvature in the human spine (fig. 2-9). Cervical pillows and rolls are designed to support "natural" curvature in

the neck or create it if it isn't there. My approach encourages you to lengthen rather than curve your cervical spine. A normal rectangular or square pillow of a thickness and firmness appropriate to the shape of your neck works best.

Only if you have significant curvature in your neck and your neck is somewhat rigid, should you use a cervical pillow (or bunch your pillow under your neck). In this case the cervical pillow is a transitional device that allows the excessively curved portion of your neck to relax against a surface rather than be unsupported. The cervical roll should never exaggerate the curvature you already have. It should have a thickness intermediate between the curvature in your neck and the ideal (little or no curvature). Over time, you will be able to reduce the thickness of the cervical roll until you don't need one any more.

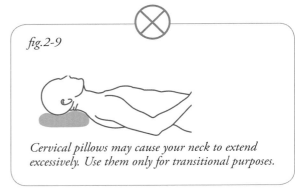
fig.2-9

Cervical pillows may cause your neck to extend excessively. Use them only for transitional purposes.

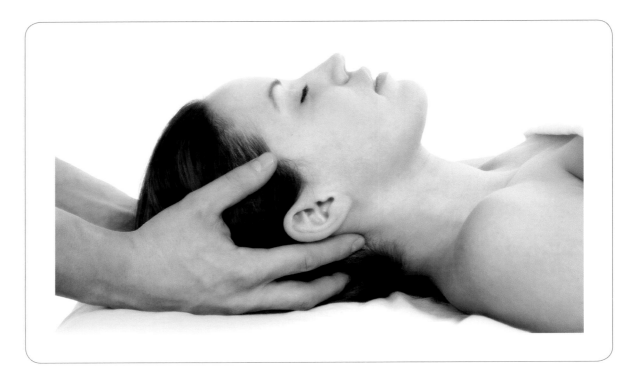

RECAP

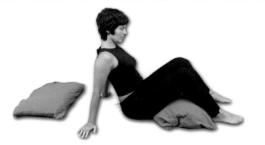

a. Bend knees

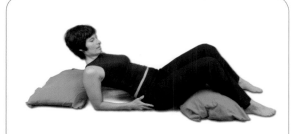

b. Lower upper body onto elbows

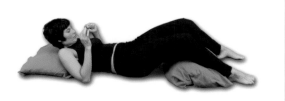

c. Unroll back onto
bed, one vertebra at a time

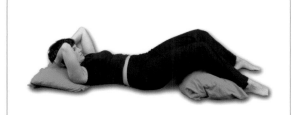

d. Lengthen back of neck

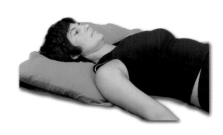

e. Press shoulders down away
from neck

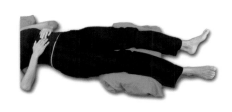

f. Straighten and relax legs, using
optional pillow beneath knees

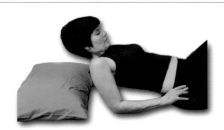

g. Check for and release an
excessive pelvic tuck

3

STACKSITTING

*Positioning your pelvis as the
foundation for your spine*

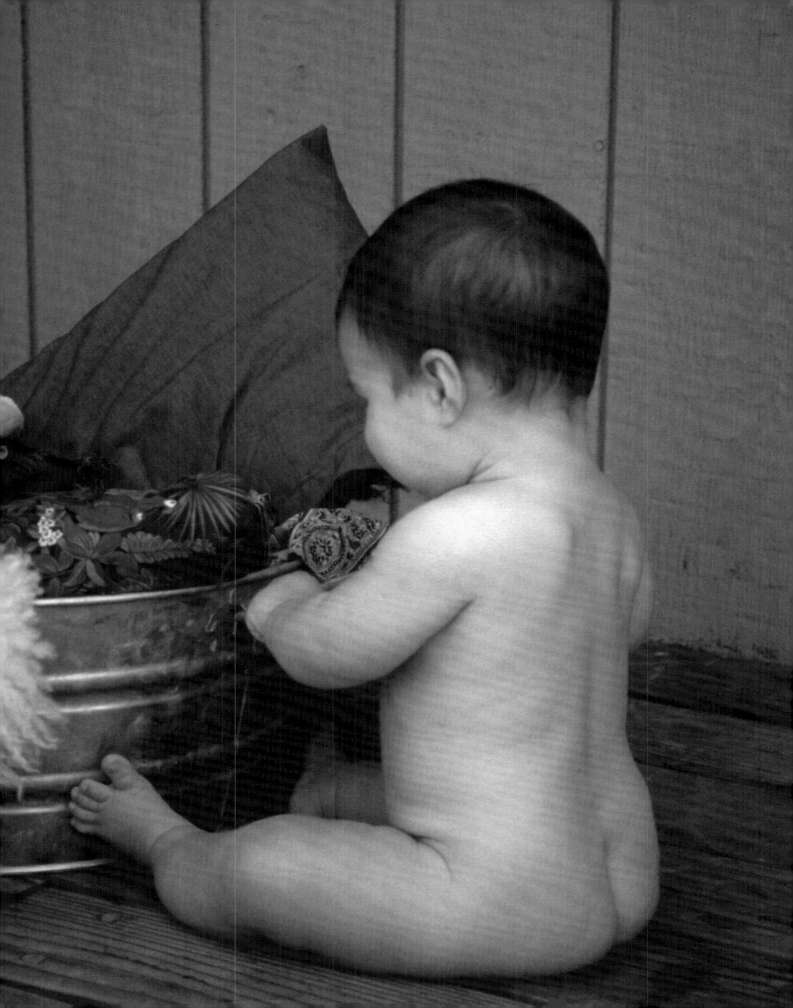

In the adjacent photographs (fig. 3-1), notice that the female rider on the left sits upright while the male rider on the right sits with a familiar slump. How would you fix the man's posture? Most people would ask him to "sit up straight," "straighten up," or pull his shoulders and neck back to be more upright. He certainly could do that, but it would require tension in his low back muscles. He would then be upright but tense, with his low back compressed and compromised. After a while, he would probably return to slumping. Many people alternate between tense muscles and a slumped back, neither of which is healthy.

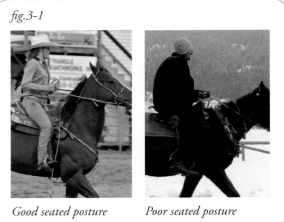

fig.3-1

Good seated posture   *Poor seated posture*

fig.3-2

The pelvis is the foundation for the upper body. With the pelvis well positioned, the upper body can be upright and relaxed. With the pelvis poorly positioned, the upper body is either relaxed but slumped, or upright but tense.

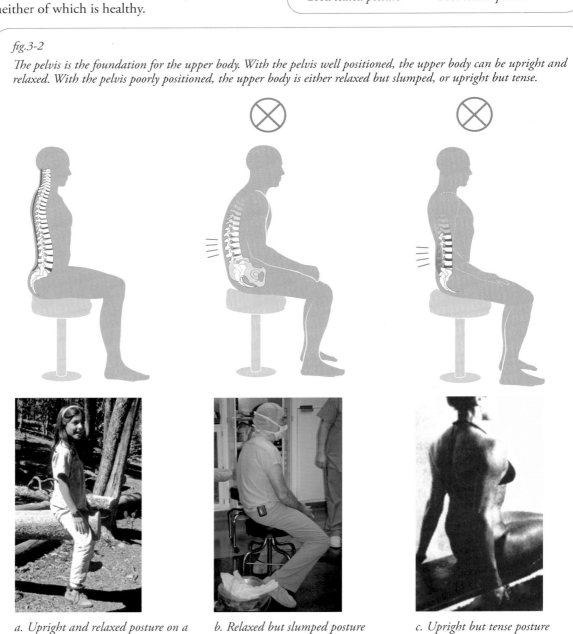

a. Upright and relaxed posture on a well-positioned (anteverted) pelvis.

b. Relaxed but slumped posture on a tucked (retroverted) pelvis.

c. Upright but tense posture on a tucked (retroverted) pelvis.

What is really needed is a shift in the pelvis at the base of the spine. This piece of our anatomy serves as the foundation for the rest of our structure. In our species, the pelvis is designed to be tipped forward (*anteverted*). When your pelvis is anteverted, the rest of your spine can stack well, so that you can be both upright and relaxed without requiring a lot of muscle tension to support your spine (fig.3-2a). When your pelvis is poorly positioned, you will be either relaxed but slumped (fig. 3-2b) or upright but tense (fig.3-2c).

One way to gauge pelvic position is to imagine that you have a tail (fig.3-3). If you look again at the picture of the two riders in fig.3-1, and imagine they both have tails, the one sitting upright would have her tail behind her, whereas the horseman who is slumping would be sitting on his tail.

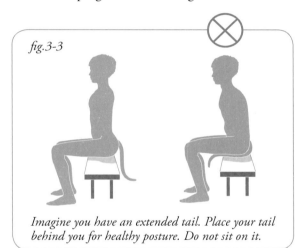

Imagine you have an extended tail. Place your tail behind you for healthy posture. Do not sit on it.

In this lesson, you will learn more about the art and science of sitting. In Lesson 1, you learned how to use a backrest to place your back in therapeutic traction as you sit. But a backrest isn't always available, and sometimes, even when one is available, it is not practical to use it (for example, when you eat). In this lesson, you will learn how to sit well without a backrest.

This lesson also lets you experience a key concept of my method. Contrary to popular belief, good posture is not something that requires a grand effort. It is, for the most part, relaxed. What it takes is the right positioning of the bones, which enables the muscles to relax. When your pelvis is well positioned, your vertebrae will stack easily with a minimum of muscle tension, like a tower of building blocks positioned on a stable foundation (fig.3-4). I call this "stacksitting."

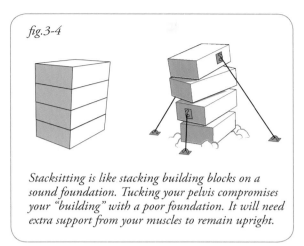

Stacksitting is like stacking building blocks on a sound foundation. Tucking your pelvis compromises your "building" with a poor foundation. It will need extra support from your muscles to remain upright.

THE WEDGE

In people who have tucked their pelvis for years, the surrounding tissues have adapted to this architecture. The muscles and ligaments in the groin area, as well as the hamstring muscles, tend to be short and tight, while the muscles in the buttocks tend to be weak and underdeveloped. To compensate for this distorted baseline position, it is helpful to sit on a wedge (fig.3-5).

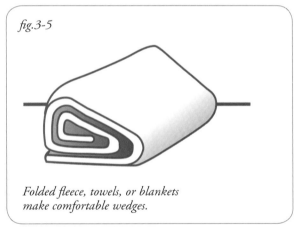

Folded fleece, towels, or blankets make comfortable wedges.

A good wedge facilitates tipping the pelvis forward (*anteversion*), and can transform your sitting experience quite dramatically (fig.3-6, fig.3-7a). You may find that your spine immediately stacks effortlessly and comfortably on its base, and you can sit for hours in one position. Especially during the period of transition, as you train your body, a wedge will compensate for the compromised structures in the pelvic area. When a wedge is not available, an alternative is to sit on the very front edge of a firm chair, allowing your pelvis to tip forward (fig.3-7b).

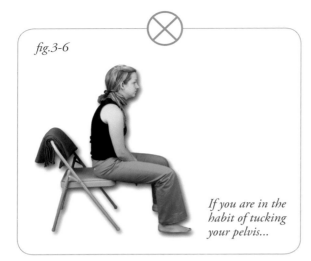

fig.3-6

If you are in the habit of tucking your pelvis...

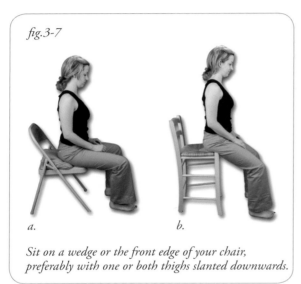

fig.3-7

a.   *b.*

Sit on a wedge or the front edge of your chair, preferably with one or both thighs slanted downwards.

THE ANTEVERTED PELVIS

When your pelvis is anteverted, your back muscles relax, which has implications far beyond comfortable sitting.

One important effect is improved breathing. With relaxed back muscles, there is an elastic movement in the spine (fig.3-8a). During inhalation, the spine lengthens. During exhalation, it settles back to its baseline length.

The new elasticity in the torso promotes good circulation, which promotes tissue health around the area of the spine, and improves overall health. Normalizing this area can have a positive effect on all of your muscles, organs, and other tissues.

This concept is so important that it bears repeating:

- The tissues around the spine remain healthy only if they have good circulation.
- Good circulation around the spine happens only if there is movement in the area.
- Nature's way of providing movement in this area is through a healthy breathing pattern.
- A healthy breathing pattern can happen only if the muscles in the area are relaxed.
- The muscles in the area can relax only if there is a sound stacking of the bones.
- And the bones stack well only if the pelvis is positioned well.

With relaxed chest (*pectoral*) muscles, breathing also causes an expansive movement in the chest (fig.3-8a). During inhalation, the sternum rises. During exhalation, it settles back to its normal position. Over a period of years, this movement increases the size of the rib cage and the capacity of the lungs.

Incidentally, you may notice that your abdomen becomes less involved in breathing, except when you need extra oxygen for cardiovascular exercise, playing wind instruments, singing, and such.

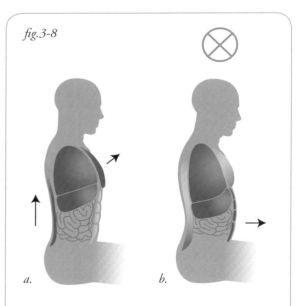

fig.3-8

a.   *b.*

a. When your back and pectoral muscles are relaxed and your abdominal muscles have good tone, your resting breathing action will be primarily in the back and chest. b. If your back and chest are tight and/or your abdominal muscles are flaccid, your resting breathing action will be mainly in the belly.

Another effect of pelvic anteversion is that your pelvic organs will be well-supported by your pubic bone (fig.3-9a). With a tucked pelvis (fig.3-9b), the main supporting structure under the pelvic organs is the rather flimsy Kegel (*pubo-coccygeal*) muscle. In my clinical experience a tucked (*retroverted*) pelvis predisposes women for organ prolapse and urinary incontinence.

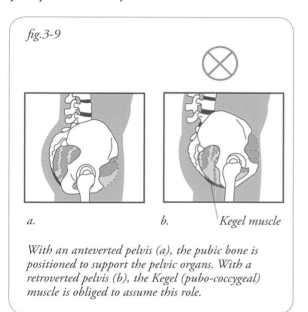

fig.3-9

a.   b.   *Kegel muscle*

With an anteverted pelvis (a), the pubic bone is positioned to support the pelvic organs. With a retroverted pelvis (b), the Kegel (pubo-coccygeal) muscle is obliged to assume this role.

By tipping the pelvis, you will also be protecting the wedge-shaped L5-S1 disc and restoring normal architecture and function to the pelvic organs.

If you are not used to this position, learning to tip your pelvis may be difficult. Stacksitting and stretchlying on your side (Lesson 4) help to cultivate the habit. The wedge or the bed "hold" your pelvis in place, so you do not have to consciously maintain this position. Proceed very slowly and gently. Initially, practice a few minutes several times a day, gradually lengthening the time as the position becomes comfortable. When not sitting with a wedge, try to maximize the time spent sitting in traction as you learned to do in Lesson 1.

Caution

If you have a diagnosis, or any suspicion, of a herniated disc in the lower lumbar area (L5-S1), it is extremely important that you not antevert your pelvis prematurely. Doing so may pinch off the herniated portion of the disc (fig.3-10). Skip this and the following lesson (Stretchlying on Your Side). Lessons 1, 2, and

5 teach you safe ways to lengthen your spine, which will make you more comfortable and can accelerate the healing of the herniated disc.

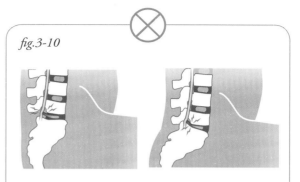

fig.3-10

Caution If you have any suspicion of a herniated disc, skip this lesson and the next because anteverting your pelvis can pinch off the herniated portion of your disc.

BENEFITS

• Allows you to sit comfortably for hours

• Relaxes back muscles

• Facilitates elastic action of breathing

• Provides strong support for pelvic organs

• Facilitates optimal circulation throughout the back

• Allows for repair and optimal function of surrounding tissues and organs

Many years ago, I had back pain. I couldn't sit on the floor for even a minute, because my back couldn't tolerate it. Now I can sit on the floor and play with my toddler. I still sit the way Esther taught me at concerts and lectures, and no longer come out with back pain or fatigue.

Jessica Davidson, M.D., Internal Medicine, Palo Alto Medical Foundation, Palo Alto, CA

EQUIPMENT

You will need the following:
- *A full-length mirror*
- *A stool or chair with a firm seat and a straight (or no) back*
- *Comfortable form-fitting clothing that permits you to evaluate the position of your pelvis and shape of your spine. Don't wear jeans, which can distort your baseline position and make it difficult to evaluate your posture.*

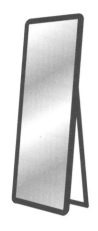

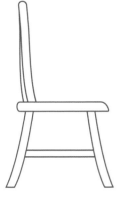

In the first part of this lesson you will analyze how you currently sit, evaluating where you need to make adjustments. In the second part, you will experiment to make those adjustments, attaining a healthy and well-aligned seated position.

EVALUATING YOUR CURRENT POSTURE

1 PLACE THE CHAIR SIDEWAYS IN FRONT OF THE MIRROR, SO THAT YOU CAN SEE YOUR BODY IN PROFILE

2 SIT ON THE FRONT OF THE CHAIR AWAY FROM THE BACKREST

Try to assume your habitual sitting posture rather than what you perceive to be correct. Your posture may resemble one of these images.

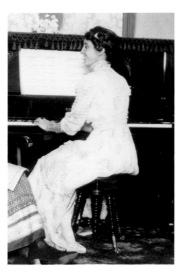

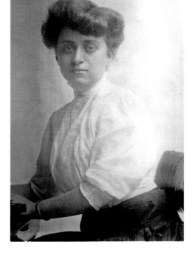

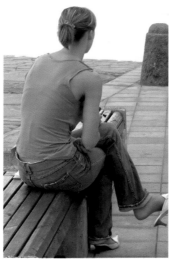

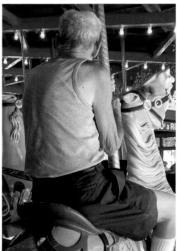

3 LOOK IN THE MIRROR TO ASSESS THE POSITION OF YOUR PELVIS

Compare the position of your pelvis with one of the sets of pictures and drawings on this page.

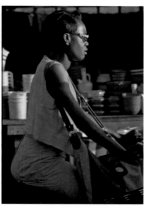

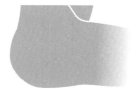

A tipped (*anteverted*) pelvis is the ideal and supports a well-stacked spine and relaxed back, neck, and shoulder muscles.

Ideal (anteverted) pelvis

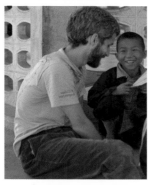

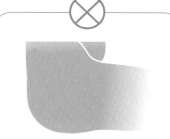

A tucked (*retroverted*) pelvis threatens the discs in the lumbar spine. It results in a forward thrust of the head and neck and, therefore, tense neck and shoulder muscles.

Tucked (retroverted) pelvis

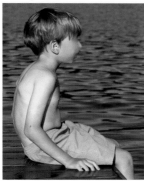

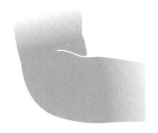

A severely tucked pelvis is an exaggerated version of a tucked pelvis, and is associated with similar problems.

Severely tucked (retroverted) pelvis

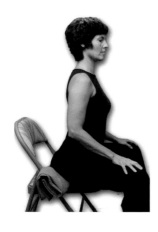

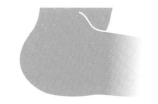

An overly tipped pelvis results in a sway and tight low back muscles. (Most people do not naturally overtip their pelvises but may do so as they try to correct a pelvic tuck.)

Overly tipped (overly anteverted) pelvis

IDEAL AND COMPROMISED LOW BACK SHAPES

4 ASSESS THE SHAPE OF YOUR LOW BACK

Compare your reflection in the mirror with one of the sets of pictures and drawings on this page.

STRAIGHT

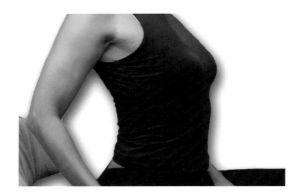

A healthy low back is relatively flat, has relaxed back muscles, and decompressed discs.

ROUNDED (KYPHOTIC)

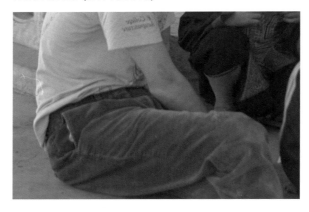

A rounded (*kyphotic*) low back causes discs to bulge posteriorly, in the direction of the spinal nerve roots.

SWAYED (LORDOTIC)

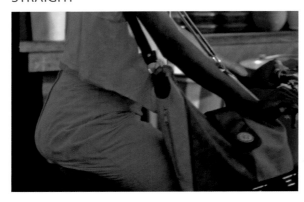

A swayed (*lordotic*) low back has tight back muscles, compromised circulation, and compressed discs.

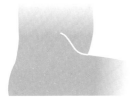

Ideal (straight) low back

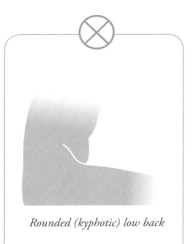

Rounded (kyphotic) low back

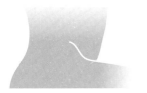

Swayed (lordotic) low back

5 WITH YOUR FINGERTIPS, ASSESS THE SPINAL GROOVE IN YOUR LOW BACK

Locate the vertical midline of the low back. Feel the individual vertebrae lying in the groove created by the long (*erector spinae*) muscles that run vertically on either side of the spine. Is the groove deep or shallow? Are the ridges on either side like a tightly drawn bowstring or do they "give" easily under pressure? As you run your fingertips up and down along the groove, does it change depth significantly?

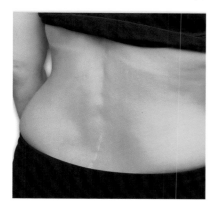

An ideal low back has a mild groove, embedded bumps (vertebrae), and soft ridges on either side of the groove.

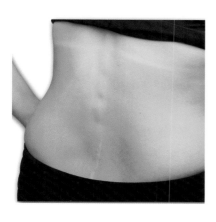

A rounded (*kyphotic*) low back has no groove, prominent bumps (vertebrae), and subtle or no ridges.

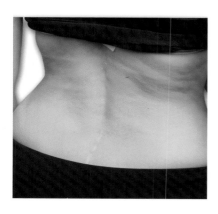

A swayed (*lordotic*) low back has a deep groove and taut muscle ridges on either side of the groove. The bumps in the midline groove are difficult to feel.

IDEAL AND PROBLEMATIC SPINAL GROOVES

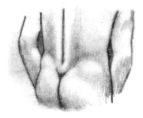

An ideal low back with mild spinal groove

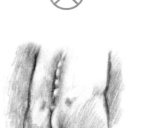

Rounded (kyphotic) low back with no groove

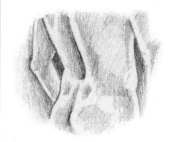

Swayed (lordotic) low back with deep groove

If you find that your pelvis is tipped, your low back is straight, your spinal groove is of even depth throughout the spine, and you sit comfortably, you are well on your way to the ideal sitting position.

You may not need to work through the first six steps of this section, starting on page 80. But take a look at them anyway, before tackling Step 7 on page 82.

EXAMPLES OF STACKSITTING

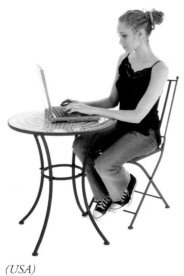

(USA)

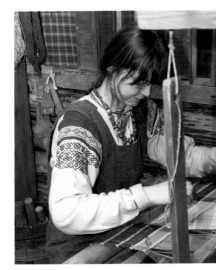

(USSR)

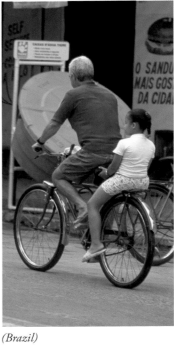

(Brazil)

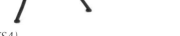

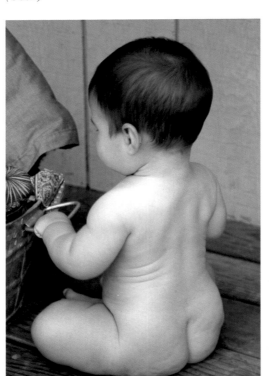

(Egypt)

(USA)

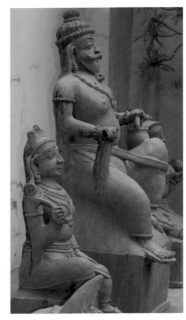

(India)

EXAMPLES OF STACKSITTING

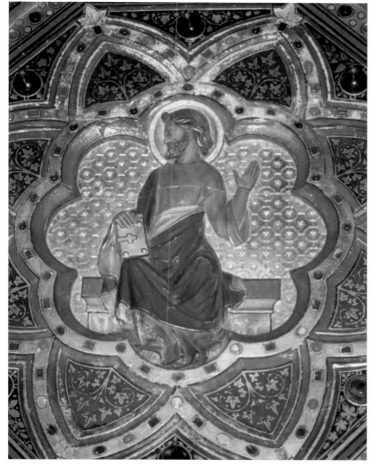

(France)

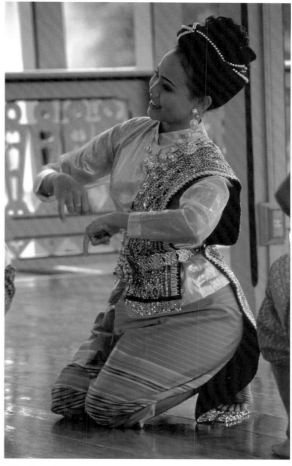

(Thailand)

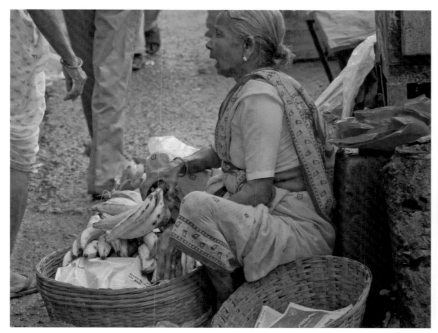

(India)

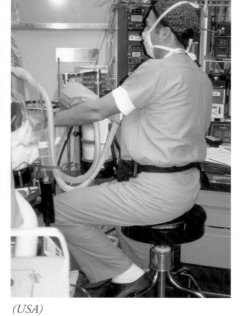

(USA)

EQUIPMENT

You will need the following:
- *A full-length mirror*
- *A stool or chair with a firm seat and a straight (or no) back*
- *A wedge for the seat of the chair*

The wedge should be made of a firm yet soft material: firm enough to provide support for the sitz bones (ischial tuberosities), yet soft enough to be comfortable. Materials that work well include small wool or fleece throws, cotton batting, flannel sheets, and towels.

To make the wedge, fold the material so that it is about as wide as the chair seat but half as deep, and significantly thicker in the back than in the front. The goal is that it be comfortable and provide a definite forward slope on which your sitz bones will rest. This slope helps your pelvis tip forward.

Most commercial wedges are too soft or too firm, don't easily adjust, and don't provide the correct forward slope.

I have developed a chair that is especially designed to help you stacksit. (To order, visit www.gokhalemethod.com)

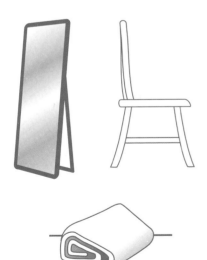

ADJUSTING YOUR SEATED POSTURE

1 PLACE A WEDGE ON THE CHAIR

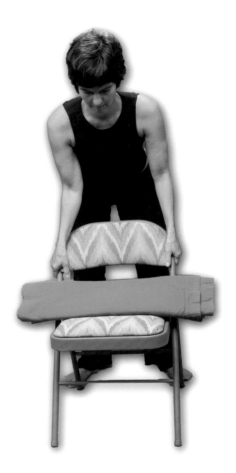

Position the wedge so it helps to tip your pelvis forward when you sit.

In situations where you cannot use a wedge, you can sit on the front edge of the chair with your thighs angled downward (see fig.3-7b on page 72).

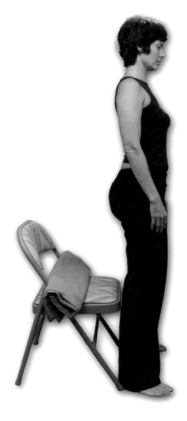

2 STAND WITH YOUR BACK TO THE CHAIR AND YOUR FEET HIP-WIDTH APART

This wide stance will help you learn to stacksit. Later, you will be able to vary your foot position and still sit well.

3 IF POSSIBLE, POSITION YOUR FEET INTO A KIDNEY-BEAN SHAPE

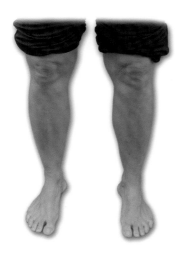

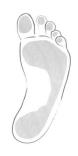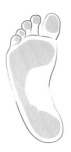

This step aligns the feet and legs optimally, but if you have trouble with it, skip it for now. You will learn more about it in a later lesson.

Kidney bean shaped feet organize the bones and soft tissue of the feet, legs, and hips optimally.

4 BEND AT YOUR HIPS AND THEN AT YOUR KNEES, LOWERING YOURSELF ONTO THE FRONT EDGE OF THE WEDGE

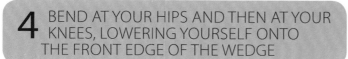

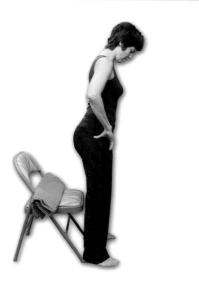

This tips your pelvis forward and settles your pelvis between your legs. It can be difficult to attain this position at first, yet you use it automatically whenever you seat yourself on a toilet. Try to recreate that position.

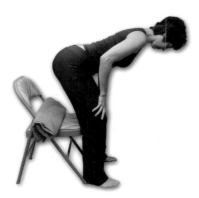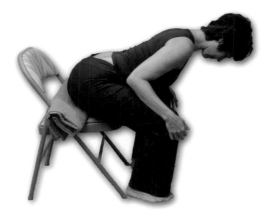

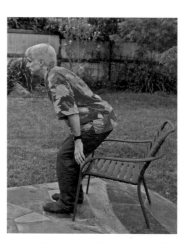

Hinging at the hip joint when beginning to sit helps position the pelvis for stacksitting (USA).

EXAMPLES OF STACKSITTING

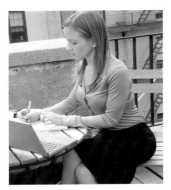

(USA)

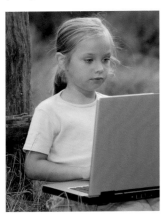

(USA)

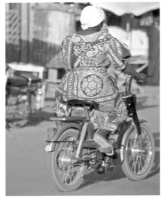

(Burkina Faso)

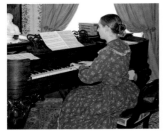

(USA)

5 ANCHOR YOUR RIB CAGE

Contract the upper abdominal muscles to pull the front of the rib cage downward and inward, thus lengthening and straightening the low back. This maneuver is difficult to learn but very important to master. Use your abdominal muscles to maintain a healthy alignment in the next three steps. If you have difficulty locating these muscles, refer to the exercise on page 198 in the Appendix 1.

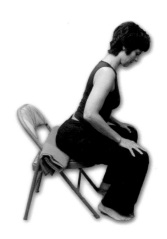

6 LEAVING YOUR PELVIS TIPPED FORWARD AND YOUR RIBCAGE ANCHORED, COME TO AN UPRIGHT POSITION

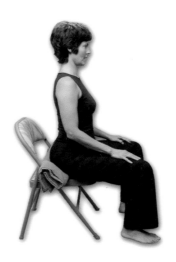

Hinge only at the hips to return to an upright position.

7 PERFORM A SHOULDER ROLL WITH EACH SHOULDER

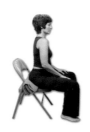 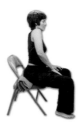 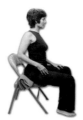 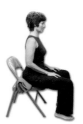

Note that the abdominal muscles work to keep the lower front rim of the ribcage anchored. In stretchsitting, the backrest prevents the low back from swaying. Here the abdominal muscles fulfill this role.

⊗

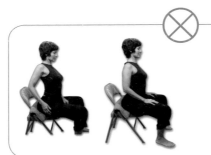

A common mistake is to move the rib cage with the shoulder, causing the low back to sway.

8 LENGTHEN YOUR NECK

Use one of the ways you learned in Lesson 1 (p.44), to lengthen your neck. Resist the tendency to sway.

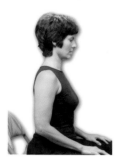

Option A
Imagine a helium balloon inside your head is trying to escape. Consciously release any tension in your neck muscles that works against the balloon's upward thrust.

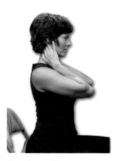

Option C
Position your fingertips in the two side indentations at the base of your skull (the *occipital grooves*) and move your skull up and away from your body.

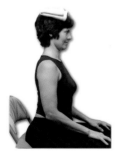

Option E
Place (or imagine) a light object on the crown of your head. Push up against it. This engages the *longus colli muscle* to help lengthen your neck.

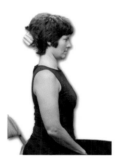

Option B
Grab a clump of hair at the base of your skull and gently pull it back and up.

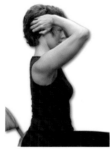

Option D
Grasp the base of your skull with both hands and gently pull toward the top of your head.

EXAMPLES OF HEALTHY NECK ALIGNMENT

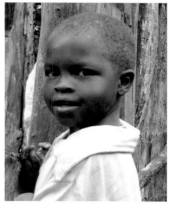

(Kenya)

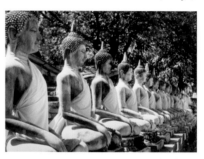

(Thailand)

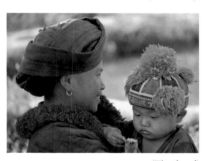

(Thailand)

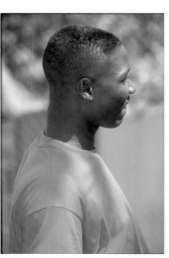

(Burkina Faso)

ART PIECES SHOWING STACKSITTING

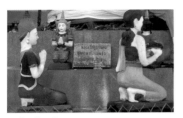

(Thailand)

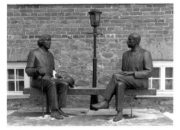

(Estonia)

THE RIB ANCHOR

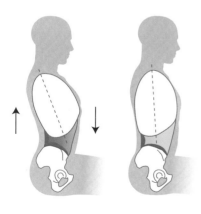

A healthy way to flatten the low back

9 COMPLETELY RELAX YOUR BODY

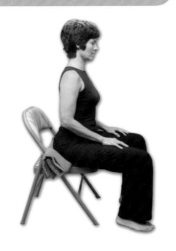

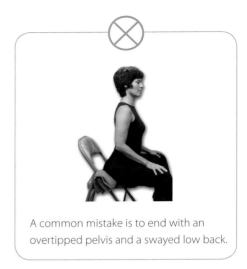

A common mistake is to end with an overtipped pelvis and a swayed low back.

Look in the mirror to see if you achieved the desirable combination of a tipped pelvis and a relatively straight low back. If so, skip to Step 14.

10 IF YOU OVERCORRECT AND YOUR PELVIS IS SEVERELY TIPPED, BACK OFF

Overtipping forces an arch into your low back. You can ease the arch by:
* Shifting your weight to the left and lifting the right buttock, then repositioning the right sitz bones slightly further forward.
* Repeating this action with the left buttock.

11 IF YOU FIND YOURSELF SWAYING, USE YOUR "RIB ANCHOR"

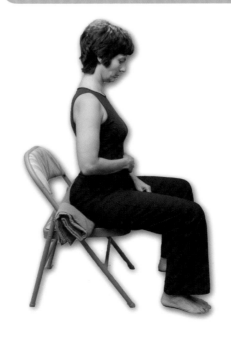

As you learned to do in Step 5, rotate the bottom front of your rib cage down and back until it aligns with the contour of your abdomen. You will be using several abdominal muscles, especially the *internal obliques*. It may help to use one of your hands to guide the movement. If you have trouble with this movement, refer to page 198 of Appendix 1 for a way to perform the movement lying on your back with the floor to guide you.

12 IF YOU FIND YOURSELF SLUMPING, YOU MAY NEED TO TIP YOUR PELVIS FURTHER FORWARD

There are several ways to correct the position of your pelvis. Begin with Option A and come upright to see if you still sway or slump. (Be sure you are not swaying because you have tipped your pelvis too far forward.) If necessary, try Option B. Continue through the options until you succeed in tipping your pelvis forward.

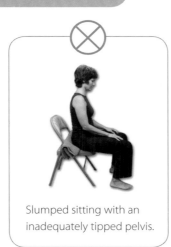

Slumped sitting with an inadequately tipped pelvis.

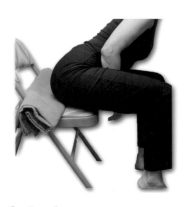 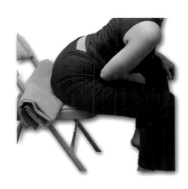

Option A
Lean forward from the hips with a straight back and rest your elbows on your thighs. Shift your weight onto your left buttock. Walk your right buttock back higher onto the wedge. Then repeat to move your left buttock higher on the wedge.

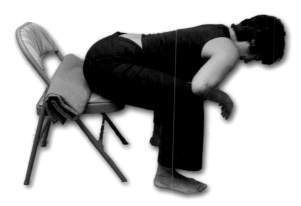

Option B
Lean forward from the hips with a straight back and rest your elbows on your knees. Lift both buttocks a little off the chair while tipping your pelvis a little further forward. Then reposition your sitz bones on the wedge.

EXAMPLES OF HEALTHY PELVIC ANTEVERSION WHEN SITTING

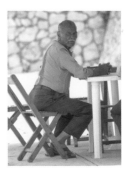

(Mexico)

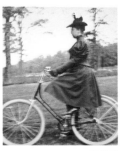

(USA)

EXAMPLES OF STACKSITTING WITH A WEDGE

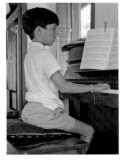

(USA)

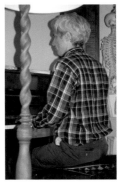

(USA)

EXAMPLES OF CHILDREN BEING CARRIED WITH GOOD PELVIC POSITIONING

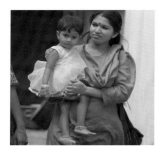

(India)

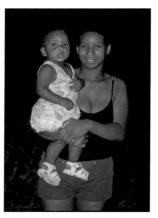

(Brazil)

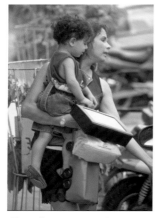

(Brazil)

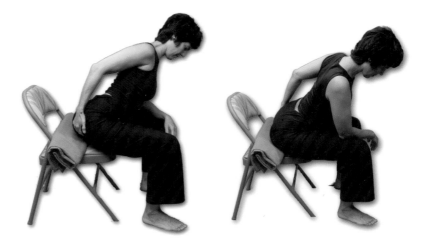

Option C
Shift your weight to your left buttock. With your right arm, reach behind and under your right buttock. Grab the flesh and pull it back as you lower the buttock onto the wedge. Repeat on the other side.

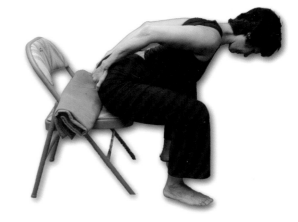

Option D
Lean forward and grab the flesh of both buttocks, Lift yourself off the chair momentarily and pull your flesh up and back. Then lower your buttocks onto the wedge.

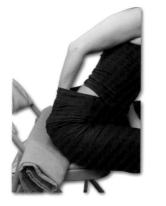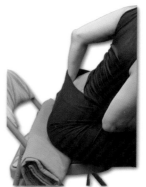

Option E
Lean forward from the hip with a straight back and rest your left elbow on your thigh. Shift your weight onto your left buttock and reach inside your pants to grasp the flesh of your right buttock. Place your right sitz bone back on the wedge. Then repeat with your left buttock. Obviously, this move is best done in private!

13 RETURN TO AN UPRIGHT POSITION, ONCE AGAIN RELAXING YOUR BODY

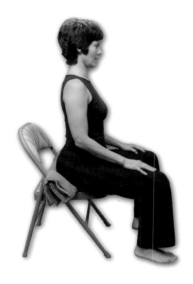

If you still find yourself slumping, begin again, using a higher wedge. You may need to experiment with different wedges until you find one that helps you attain the optimum sitting position.

14 ROLL YOUR SHOULDERS BACK AND LENGTHEN YOUR NECK

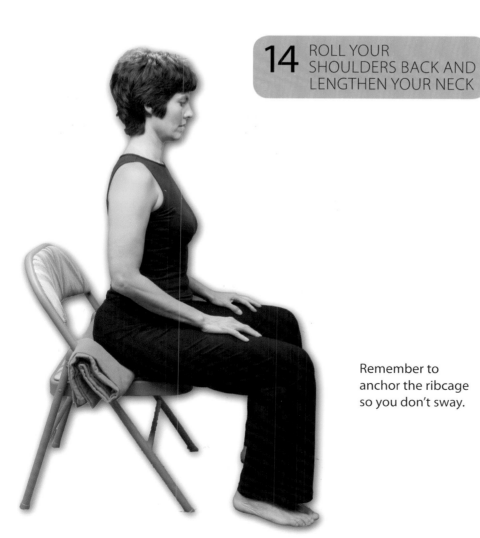

Remember to anchor the ribcage so you don't sway.

EXAMPLES OF CHILDREN STACKSITTING

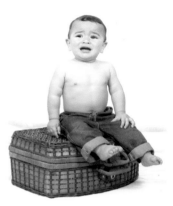

(USA)

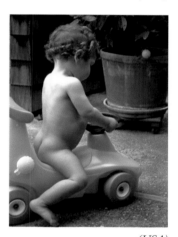

(USA)

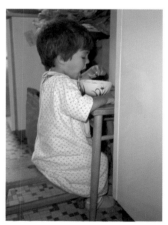

(USA)

INDICATIONS OF IMPROVEMENT

As your muscles and ligaments adjust to your new pelvic alignment, you will become more comfortable stacksitting, and will be able to sit with ease for longer periods.

When you have adopted a more upright, relaxed posture, you will notice your breathing pattern improves, increasing lung capacity and promoting good circulation.

TROUBLESHOOTING

PAIN IN THE LOW BACK
If performing any of these movements causes pain, or makes pain worse, stop immediately. Proceed to Lesson 5, where you will learn to maintain length in your spine. After mastering that, return here.

SORENESS IN THE LOW BACK
If stacksitting is a significant change from your normal sitting position and feels uncomfortable, try a position that is intermediate between your old way of sitting and the ideal. Move in the direction of the ideal, but don't expect to achieve it the first time you try.

If you have misused your back in the past, your body has learned adaptive protective mechanisms, such as pain, muscle contraction, and inflammation. Pain inhibits recklessness, muscle contraction restricts mobility (preventing further damaging motions), and inflammation hastens healing. Now that you are changing the way you move, you no longer need these layers of protection, but it takes some time for your body to adapt. Continue to practice your altered, improved posture habits until your brain perceives that the area is no longer subject to repeated misuse or threat, and it will gradually adjust the instructions it sends to the low back. Treat the area gently. Try comforting treatments, such as massage and hot baths, to coax your back into relaxation. Or consider acupuncture to "reset" the area, normalizing electrical messages between the brain and the body.

WEDGE NOT AVAILABLE
You can improvise a wedge with a folded sweater or jacket, or in a pinch, the edge of a bag or shoe (fig.3-11). Or, as mentioned earlier, use the front edge of the chair as a wedge (fig.3-7b). Allowing at least one thigh to slant downwards helps you achieve pelvic anteversion which, in turn, facilitates good alignment throughout the upper body. Sometimes people think they can simulate the effect of a wedge by thrusting their buttocks behind them, but if you have been tucking your pelvis for most of your life, your body architecture has adapted to this alignment. If you try to antevert your pelvis without a wedge, you will likely sway your low back, at least in the beginning stages of training. After some time, the baseline position of your pelvis will settle in a healthy alignment without any external help.

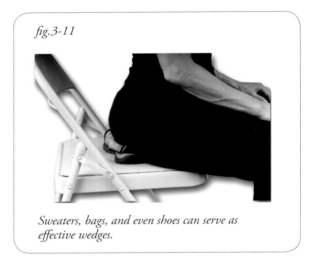

fig.3-11

Sweaters, bags, and even shoes can serve as effective wedges.

INELEGANT MOVEMENT
A forward bend as you sit down helps antevert your pelvis and minimizes pressure on the knees, but it's not always pretty. Some people are unhappy thrusting their buttocks backward and bending forward as they sit. For a more elegant series of movements, try placing one foot slightly behind the other and under the chair (fig.3-12). Then lower yourself directly onto the chair by bending mainly with your knees. Just before you sit, thrust your pelvis backward (though this will create a momentary sway). As soon as you relax onto the chair, you will no longer have the sway. This technique will give you the necessary pelvic anteversion without bending your whole body forward to attain it.

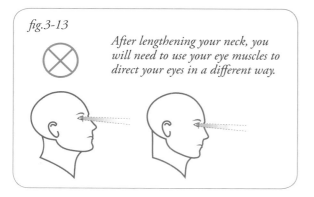

fig.3-12

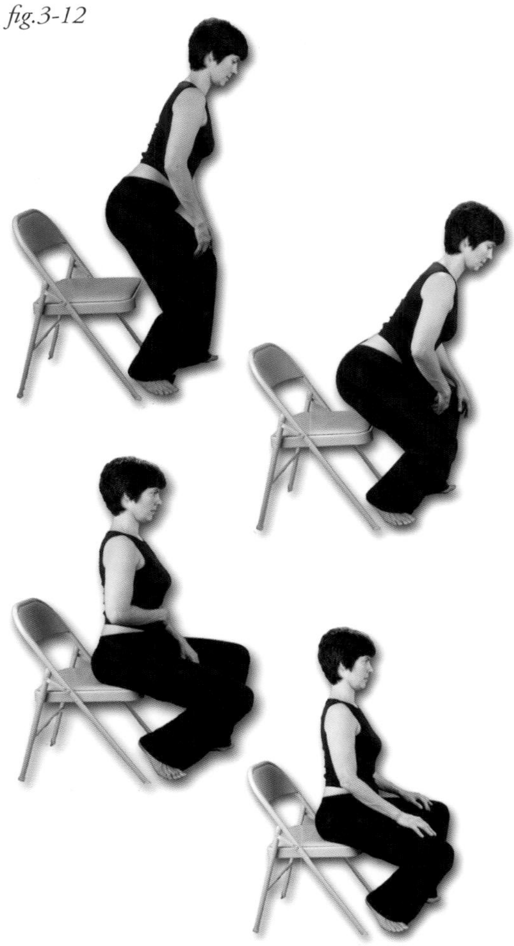

For a more elegant approach to stacksitting, actively tip the pelvis forward just momentarily.

CHANGED LINE OF VISION

When you lengthen the back of your neck, your head naturally rotates slightly downward. This downward tilt changes your line of vision, and you may find that you gaze toward the floor. Rather than distorting your neck to look straight ahead, simply raise your eyes (fig.3-13).

fig.3-13

After lengthening your neck, you will need to use your eye muscles to direct your eyes in a different way.

FURTHER INFORMATION

CONFLICTING GUIDELINES

Allowing for healthy anteversion in the pelvis is perhaps the most basic and far-reaching postural measure you will learn, but I realize these guidelines may be in direct conflict with what you have been taught elsewhere. Current medical and lay thinking still encourage a tucked, retroverted pelvis. Yet this compresses the anterior portion of the wedge-shaped L5-S1 disc, compromising its integrity (fig.F-25 on page 21). It also leads to numerous other distortions throughout the musculo-skeletal and organ systems (fig.3-2 on page 70). Follow my guidelines as an experiment; then, evaluate how they work for you.

DISTINCTION BETWEEN TIPPING THE PELVIS AND SWAYING THE BACK

Some people confuse a healthy, forward-tipped pelvis with an unhealthy sway in the back. There is an important distinction. Swaying the back forms a curve in the upper lumbar area, while anteverting the pelvis creates a curve in the lower lumbar area (fig.3-14). Swaying the back is indeed unhealthy; restoring the natural arch at L5-S1 is crucial to healthy posture.

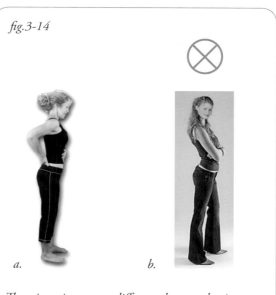

fig.3-14

a.   *b.*

There is an important difference between having a healthy lumbo-sacral arch (a), where the lower lumbar spine has significant curvature and the upper lumbar spine is relatively flat, and an unhealthy swayback (b), where the lumbo-sacral angle is small and the upper lumbar spine has significant curvature.

CHAIRS

A good chair should permit you to stretchsit or stacksit or, preferably, both. Many commercial chairs induce a pelvic tuck and/or hunched shoulders and are not conducive to healthy sitting (fig.3-15). Avoid a chair with a low seat if you have tight hamstrings and/or tight external hip rotator muscles, as it will cause you to tuck your pelvis and therefore distort your alignment. Avoid a chair so high that your legs dangle above the floor, as it may distort your back (fig.3-16). If your chair does not support you well, sit on the edge, allowing your pelvis to tip forward and your thighs to angle downward (fig.3-17).

I am often asked if the Danish kneeling chairs are conducive to good posture. For people who use them well, these chairs can provide a good option for short periods of time, because the forward-tilted seat encourages pelvic anteversion. However, when not used well, the tilted seat can also contribute to a significant sway in the low back. Settling one's weight on the knee rest for prolonged periods can also put excessive pressure on the knee and hip joints (as the thigh bone pushes into the hip socket).

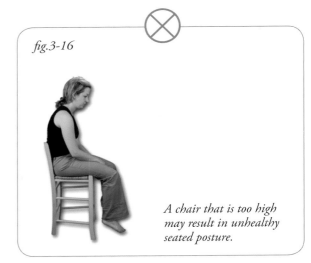

fig.3-16

A chair that is too high may result in unhealthy seated posture.

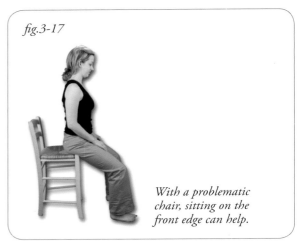

fig.3-17

With a problematic chair, sitting on the front edge can help.

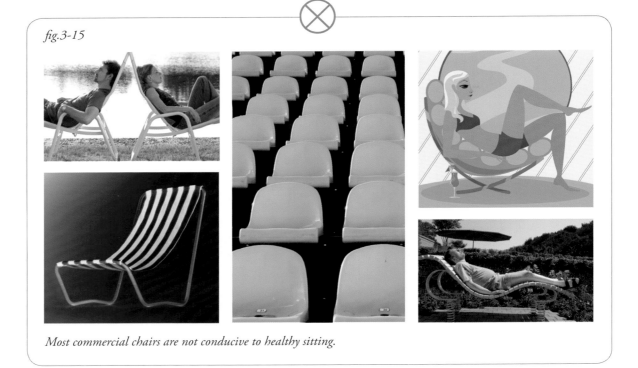

fig.3-15

Most commercial chairs are not conducive to healthy sitting.

FLOOR

Sitting on the floor causes most Westerners to either tuck their pelvis and round their low back, or sway to be upright (fig.3-18). This is because the necessary flexibility to sit well on the floor is rare in the West.

If your hamstrings and external hip rotator muscles are extremely flexible, you may be able to sit on the floor and still preserve your pelvic anteversion (fig.3-19).

When you do sit on the floor (for example, to play with small children), it is advisable to use a sitting cushion like the traditional Japanese zafu or a low bench (fig.3-20a). If your knees are healthy, you can sit with your buttocks resting on your heels in the Japanese "seiza" position (fig.3-20b). Another alternative is to use one or both arms to prop you up and lengthen your spine (fig.3-20c).

fig.3-20

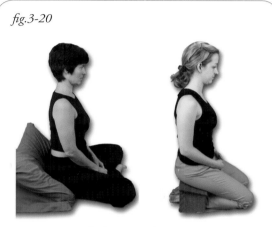

a. Using a prop facilitates stacksitting on the floor.

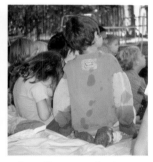

b. Sitting in the Japanese "seiza" position facilitates stacksitting, but requires healthy knees.

fig.3-18

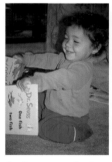

a. Tucking the pelvis and rounding the low back when sitting on the floor

b. Swaying the back when sitting upright on the floor

Sitting cross-legged on the floor unaided is problematic for most people in modern industrialized societies.

fig.3-19

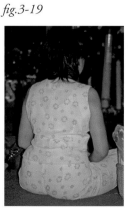

Stacksitting cross-legged on the floor unaided requires a high degree of hip flexibility (Thailand).

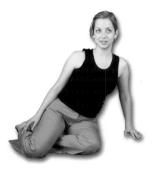

c. Using the arms to lengthen the spine facilitates sitting on the floor.

These are some healthy options for sitting on the floor.

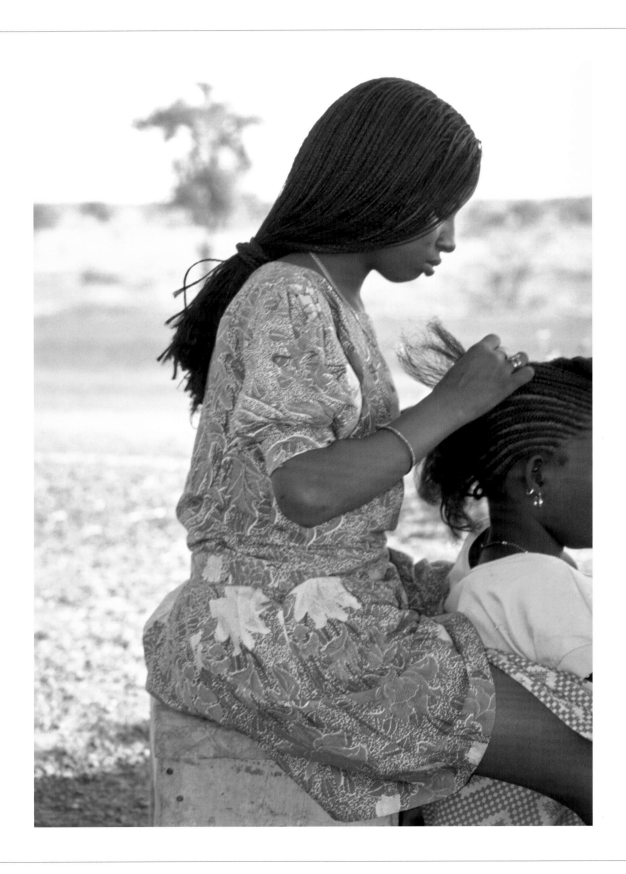

RECAP

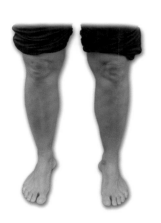

a. **Form a kidney-bean shape with each foot; rotate feet and legs outwards; allow pelvis to settle**

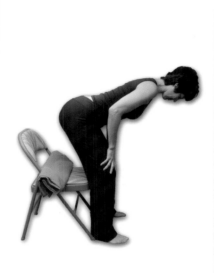

b. **Tip pelvis forward and hinge forward at hips**

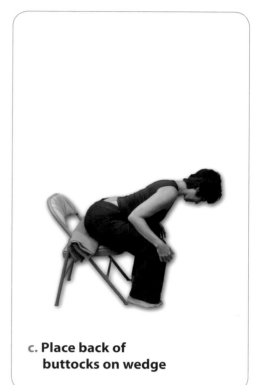

c. **Place back of buttocks on wedge**

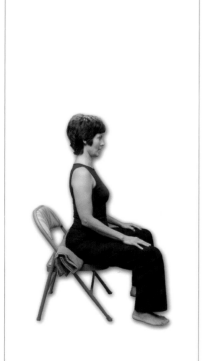

d. **Stack spine comfortably**

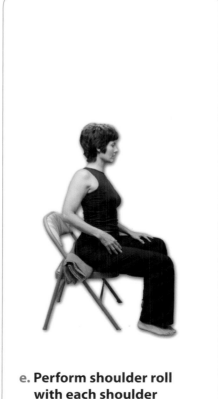

e. **Perform shoulder roll with each shoulder**

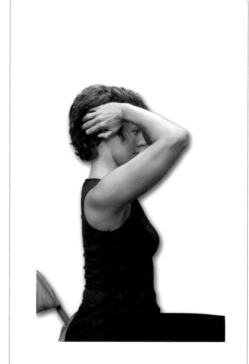

f. **Lengthen back of neck**

4

STRETCHLYING ON YOUR SIDE

Lying with a lengthened back

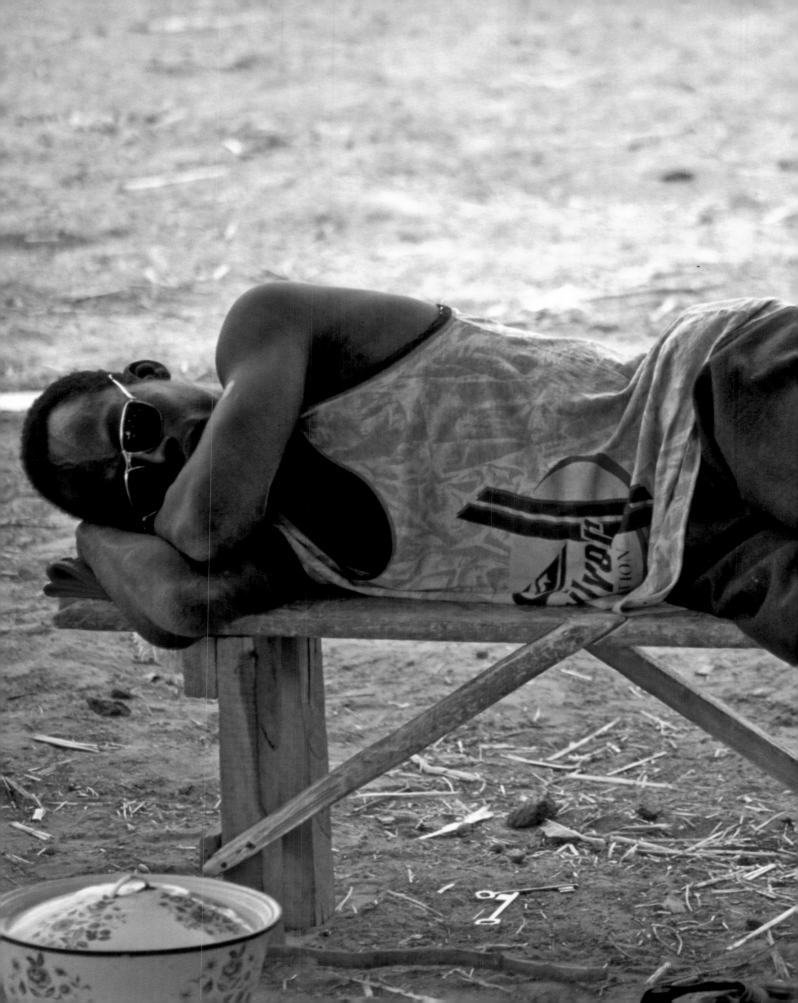

In Lesson 2, you learned a healthy way to lie on your back that also puts your spine in gentle traction. In this chapter you will learn another healthy, restful, and therapeutic sleep position: stretchlying on your side. Many people are forced to sleep on their side to reduce sleep apnea, snoring, or joint pain, and there is nothing wrong with this. Anthropological research indicates that for most of human history, it is very likely that our ancestors slept on their sides. This position allows members of a family to nest into each other for warmth, safety, and economy of ground space and cover. People living in much of the world today still tend to sleep on their sides (fig.4-1). It is certainly a natural position for us, one that we adapted to over millions of years.

fig.4-1

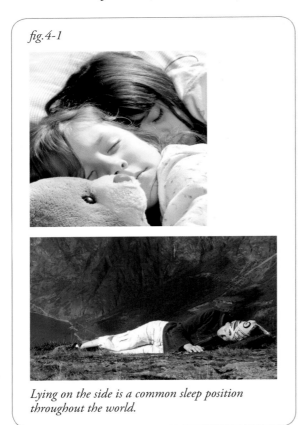

Lying on the side is a common sleep position throughout the world.

One problem is that many people who sleep on their sides assume a fetal position in which they curl their spine forward into a "C" shape (fig. 4-2a). The hunched "C" shape compresses the anterior part of the discs, forcing the contents of the discs (*nucleosus pulposum*) backwards and putting pressure on the fibrous exterior (*annular fibrosis*), causing it to fray over time (fig.4-2b). This hunched posture, if carried over to standing or sitting, is a major contributor to disc wear and tear.

fig.4-2

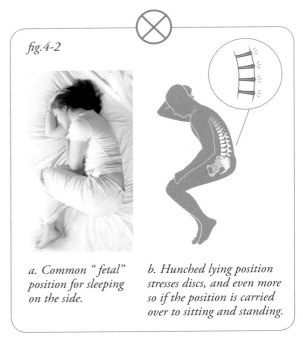

a. Common "fetal" position for sleeping on the side.

b. Hunched lying position stresses discs, and even more so if the position is carried over to sitting and standing.

fig.4-3

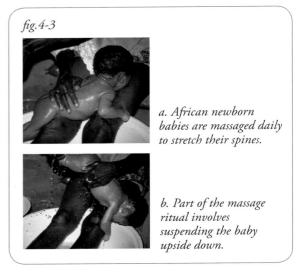

a. African newborn babies are massaged daily to stretch their spines.

b. Part of the massage ritual involves suspending the baby upside down.

Your fetal days are over! It is time to stretch yourself out and lengthen your spine. In many African countries, newborn babies are massaged and lengthened every day by a woman specializing in this care (fig.4-3a). The massage ritual goes so far as holding the baby upside down by the ankles to lengthen it (fig. 4-3b), though I do not have enough information and experience to recommend this.

Another problem is that some people who habitually sway their low backs carry this through into their side-sleeping position (fig. 4-4a). The *erector spinae* muscles on either side of the spine remain tense, reducing circulation in the area and compressing the spinal discs (fig. 4-4b).

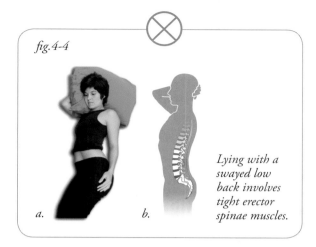

fig. 4-4

a. b.

Lying with a swayed low back involves tight erector spinae muscles.

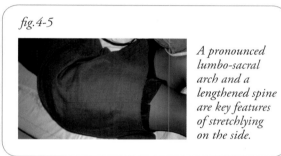

fig. 4-5

A pronounced lumbo-sacral arch and a lengthened spine are key features of stretchlying on the side.

In this chapter you will learn to lie on your side with a pronounced lumbo-sacral arch and lengthened back (fig. 4-5). This supports the health of your spinal discs, your nerve roots, and your other spinal tissues.

The proper position is not only comfortable; it is therapeutic. Lying in a neutral position helps the muscles in the area normalize to longer baseline lengths, improving circulation, which speeds healing. You lengthen your spine just as you do when sleeping on your back, and derive similar benefits.

Initially, the new position may seem awkward, but soon your body will adapt and you will enjoy restful sleep that is also therapeutic. Lying on your side offers a third way to put your back in gentle traction for many hours, complementing the benefits described in Lessons 1 and 2.

In addition, the position reinforces the practice of tipping the pelvis forward (anteversion). One immediate benefit from this maneuver is to soften the groin crease, improving the circulation to the legs and feet. You may notice your feet are warmer as they benefit from improved blood supply.

Even if you normally sleep on your back, we encourage you to work through this lesson. It is always useful to be able to sleep well in more than one healthy position, in case you are forced to give up your usual position because of injury, pregnancy, or some other cause.

Caution

For some people, the movements taught in this lesson constitute a major shift from their current posture. If you are one of these people, proceed very slowly and gently. Move in the direction of the ideal, but don't expect to achieve it the first time you try. **If you find that performing any of these movements exaggerates your pain, stop immediately.** Proceed to Lesson 5, which will help you maintain length in your spine. After mastering that technique, return here.

If you have a diagnosis, or any suspicion, of a herniated disc in the lower lumbar area (L5-S1), it is extremely important that you not antevert your pelvis prematurely. Doing so may pinch off the herniated portion of the disc (fig. 3-10 on page 73). Skip this lesson for now. Lessons 1, 2, and 5 teach you safe ways to lengthen your spine, which will make you more comfortable and can accelerate healing of the herniated disc.

BENEFITS

• Normalizes muscles to longer baseline lengths

• Decompresses discs and spinal nerve roots

• Promotes improved circulation and hastens healing

• Improves quality of sleep

• Creates muscle memory for an anteverted pelvis and a lengthened spine

Learning to stretchlie was a phenomenal breakthrough, although remarkably simple.

Charles Bacon,
Senior Research Geologist, USGS,
Menlo Park, CA

EQUIPMENT

You will need the following:
- One or more pillows to place under your head
- Possibly a pillow or wedge to place between your knees
- Possibly a small towel roll to place beneath your waist

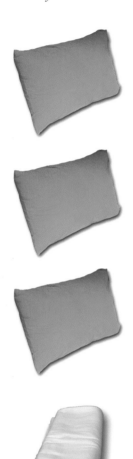

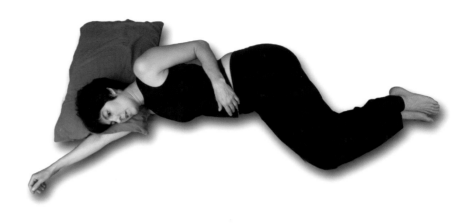

1 LIE ON YOUR SIDE IN BED AS YOU CUSTOMARILY DO

Have a few extra pillows within reach.

2 POSITION YOUR PELVIS: LIFT YOUR HIPS OFF THE BED AND TIP YOUR PELVIS FORWARD INTO ANTEVERSION

You will sense that your buttocks are thrust back with a deep crease in your groin. Note that this may cause a sway in the low back, which you will remove in the next steps.

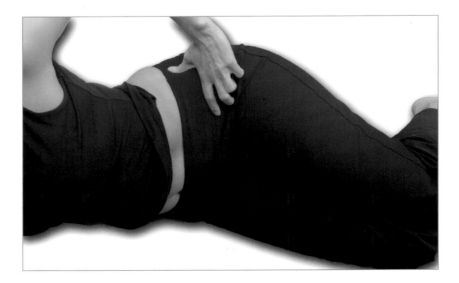

3 POSITION YOUR ARMS TO GIVE YOU LEVERAGE. THEN USE YOUR ARMS TO HOIST YOUR UPPER BODY JUST OFF THE BED

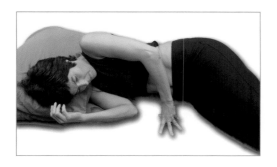

Leave your hips anchored on the bed and keep your legs relaxed. Engage your abdominal muscles just enough to prevent swaying your low back.

Push downwards with both arms to elongate the spine.

4 PUSH YOUR UPPER BODY UP AND AWAY FROM YOUR LOWER BODY USING BOTH ARMS TO LENGTHEN YOUR LOW BACK

To get an effective stretch, the direction of the push is important. It may help to visualize a bar at chest height that you are curving up and around, and to feel your belly moving backwards toward your spine.

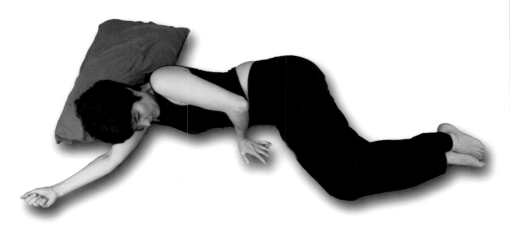

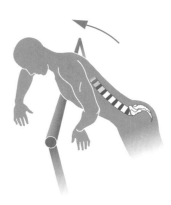

Imagine a bar that runs across the body at chest height to help you push in the right direction.

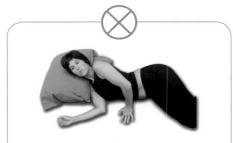

A common mistake is to arch the back while trying to lengthen it.

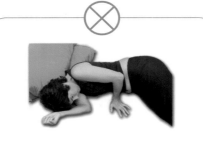

Another common mistake is to tuck the pelvis while lengthening the back.

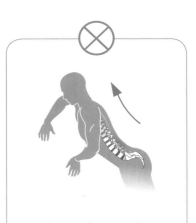

Pushing in the wrong direction may cause the low back to sway.

ZIGZAG SHAPE

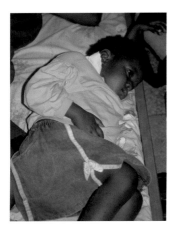

Young girl resting (Burkina Faso)

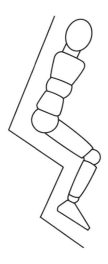

Body forms even zigzags with angles of approximately 120°

5 LAY YOUR LENGTHENED TORSO BACK ON THE BED

If you left your hips anchored to the bed, straightening your low back correctly will result in your upper body lying further forward on the bed than usual.

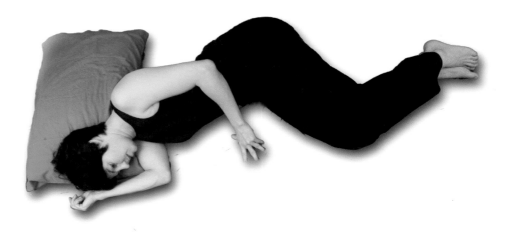

6 ASSESS YOUR OVERALL BODY SHAPE

Ideally, your lower body will form even zigzags, with approximately 120° angles at the groin, knees, and ankles.

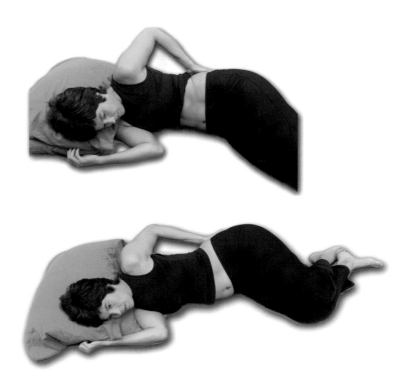

7 IF NECESSARY, REPOSITION YOUR LEGS

If your knees are too raised (towards the chest), your hamstrings may be challenged, causing your pelvis to tuck. Lowering your knees allows your pelvis to tip forward.

If your legs are too straight, your psoas muscles may be challenged, causing your low back to sway. Increasing the bend in your knees allows for slack in the psoas muscle and a lengthened lumbar spine.

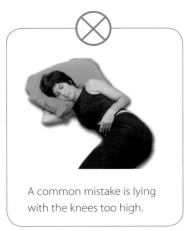

A common mistake is lying with the knees too high.

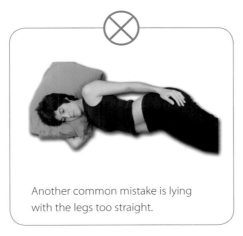

Another common mistake is lying with the legs too straight.

8 IF YOUR LOW BACK IS ROUNDED, TIP YOUR PELVIS FURTHER FORWARD

To tip pelvis further forward, raise your hips slightly off the bed. With your upper arm, reach back and around to grab your buttocks. Pull the flesh backwards and upwards to adjust your pelvis as you lower your hip onto the bed. You may need to tense your low back muscles as you do this, but later you will release that tension.

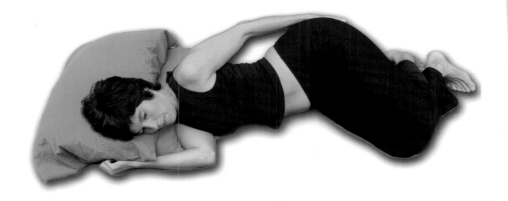

KNEES SHOULD NOT BE TOO HIGH OR TOO STRAIGHT

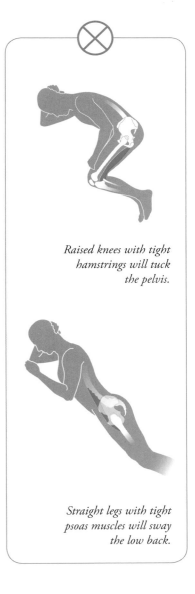

Raised knees with tight hamstrings will tuck the pelvis.

Straight legs with tight psoas muscles will sway the low back.

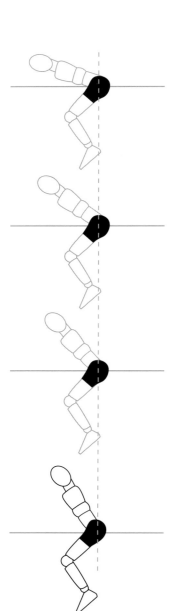

Starting from a diagonal position and swiveling the upper body backwards around the hips can help the pelvis tip forward.

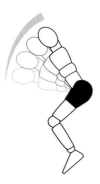

9 IF YOUR LOW BACK IS STILL ROUNDED, TIP YOUR PELVIS EVEN FURTHER FORWARD

To do this, lie diagonally on the bed. Lift your lower hip off the bed and tip your pelvis forward into anteversion. Next, keeping the pelvis pinned to the bed, use your arms to walk your upper body back. You have shifted your upper body back relative to your pelvis, resulting in a better pelvic tilt.

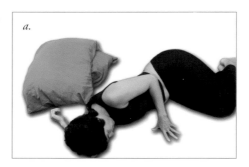
a.

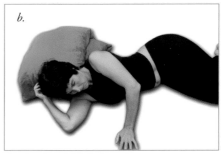
b.

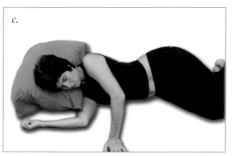
c.

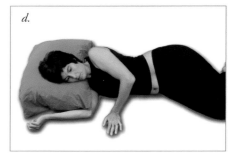
d.

10 IF YOUR LOW BACK IS SWAYED, LENGTHEN IT WHILE RETAINING THE PELVIC TILT

With your upper arm, reach around your front to your opposite side. Place your hand at the bottom of your rib cage. With your fingers, press the skin back and up, encouraging the rib cage to rotate forward. This is similar to anchoring your rib cage and lengthens your low back.

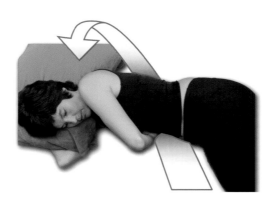

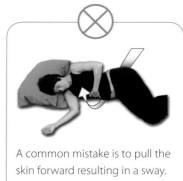

A common mistake is to pull the skin forward resulting in a sway.

11 POSITION YOUR HEAD ON A PILLOW

You may need to use more than one pillow to accommodate the width of your lower shoulder.

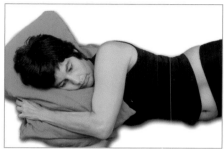

Head higher than horizontal

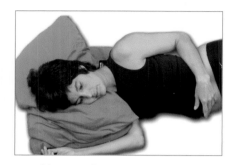

Head horizontal

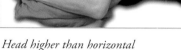

Be sure your head does not angle down, which will compromise your subsequent shoulder positioning.

12 LENGTHEN YOUR NECK

Raise your head slightly off the pillow and glide your head back and up to lengthen the back of your neck. It may be useful to grasp the hair at the base of your skull and then gently pull back and up toward your crown. Be moderate in this action. A slight stretch is comfortable and encourages your muscles to stretch and relax; a severe or sudden stretch may cause your muscles to tighten and spasm.

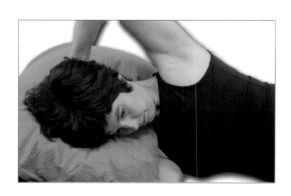

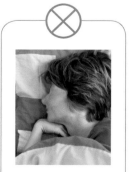

A common mistake is to raise the chin, causing compression in the neck (cervical spine).

STRETCHLYING WITH THE HEAD HIGHER THAN HORIZONTAL

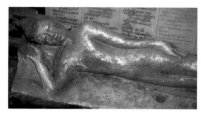

(Thailand)

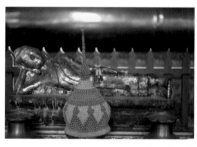

(Thailand)

All reclining Buddha images show the Buddha's head slightly elevated from the horizontal. This position is particularly healthful as it provides ample slack in the upper trapezius, facilitating good shoulder positioning.

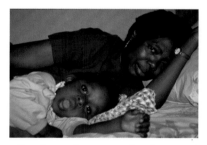

Family members resting (Burkina Faso)

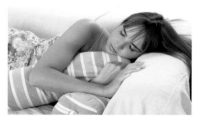

(USA)

THE UPPER SHOULDER DOES NOT SLUMP

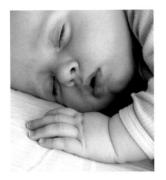

Baby sleeping (USA)

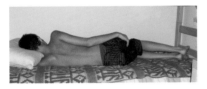

Boy lying down (USA)

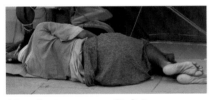

Man sleeping on street (India)

Having the shoulder rolled back allows the brachial plexus to function properly, ensuring good circulation to and from the arm. It also reduces the stress on the thoracic spine. In addition, good shoulder position when sleeping helps you become accustomed to healthy shoulder position during your waking hours.

13 PERFORM A SHOULDER ROLL WITH YOUR UPPER SHOULDER

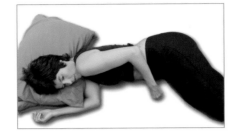

Bring your upper shoulder slightly forward, then slightly up toward your neck, and then back and down.

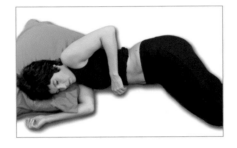

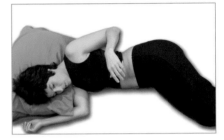

14 POSITION YOUR UPPER ARM

Here are several healthy options for positioning your upper arm in a way that prevents your upper shoulder from rounding forward.

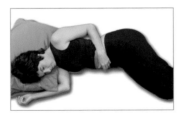

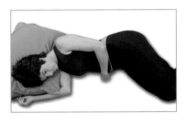

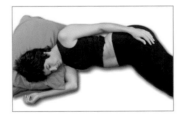

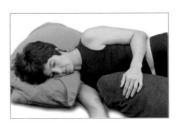

⊗

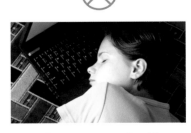

Don't allow your upper shoulder to roll forward. This stresses the upper thoracic spine and reinforces the bad habit of slumping.

15 POSITION YOUR LOWER ARM FOR COMFORT

You might try placing your lower arm in front of your body, behind your body, or under or above the head.

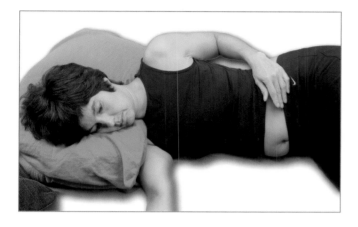

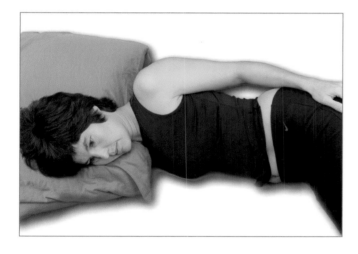

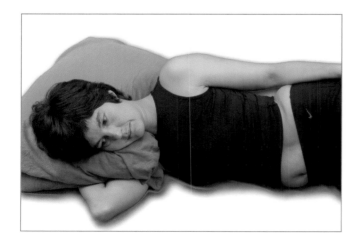

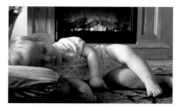

(USA)

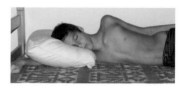

(USA)

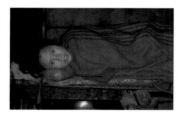

(Thailand)

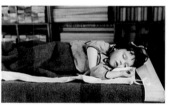

(USA)

INDICATIONS OF IMPROVEMENT

As with stretchlying on your back, stretchlying on your side may seem awkward at first. Soon you will find that you move into the position quickly and easily, and find it comfortable.

Stretchlying on your side provides the same benefits as stretchlying on your back: improved circulation, and decompression of discs and nerves. All these benefits contribute to increased comfort, function, and general well-being.

You will probably notice changes in your breathing pattern. The stretched abdominal muscles offer some resistance to belly breathing, resulting in more movement in your chest and less in your abdomen. Over time, this increase in chest breathing will expand your lung capacity and support normal architecture in your rib cage.

If you spend much of the night stretchlying, either on your back or side, the resting length of your back will increase, you will become measurably taller, and you will be more comfortable even when not in traction.

TROUBLESHOOTING

YOU CAN'T FALL ASLEEP

You may need to train your body to use this new sleeping position. Try doing some breathing meditation or perform a *body scan* (see Glossary). If some time after assuming your stretchlying position, you are still awake, revert to a more familiar position to fall asleep. As the position becomes more familiar over time, one night you will probably fall asleep. Eventually your body becomes so used to being comfortable and pain-free that it gravitates to this and other healthy positions even during sleep.

YOUR BODY DOESN'T HOLD THE POSITION THROUGH THE NIGHT

Don't worry about this! It is normal to change positions during the night. When you start the night with your back in a lengthened position, you will derive some benefit all night long. Your back muscles will remain slightly stretched, allowing for better circulation, nerve function, and disc rehydration.

YOU ARE UNCOMFORTABLE IN THIS POSITION

Elongating your spine and tipping your pelvis are difficult skills to learn. Go through the instructions again. Repeating the movements makes them more familiar and helps increase your mastery.

You may require a more perfectly neutral (straight) spine, perhaps because of a recent back injury or a significantly narrower waist than hips. If your back is healthy and you lengthen your back as you lie down, a slight sag or twist at the waist will not cause any problem. If, however, your discs are compressed, the additional pressure from sagging or twisting may cause discomfort. Try one of these suggestions:

- Place a small pillow or towel roll between your waist and the bed (fig.4-6). This eliminates the sag in the waist that results if your hips are much wider than your waist. Use the support until your back normalizes.

- Place a pillow between your knees or thighs (fig.4-7). This eliminates the twist in your back that results from your hips being wider than your knees. Use this support until your back normalizes.

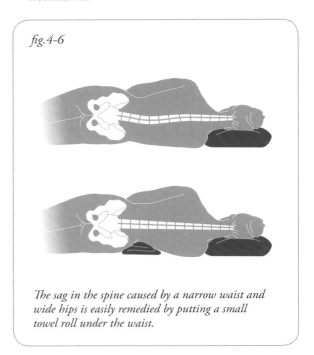

fig.4-6

The sag in the spine caused by a narrow waist and wide hips is easily remedied by putting a small towel roll under the waist.

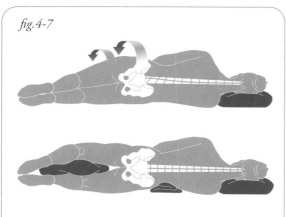

The twist in the spine caused by being narrower at the knees than at the hips when lying on the side is easily remedied with a pillow between the knees.

FURTHER INFORMATION

SLEEPING ON YOUR STOMACH

Although many people opt to sleep on their stomachs, this position can present problems. First, an ordinary pillow imposes nearly a 90° angle on the neck, which can stress or damage it. To make stomach sleeping healthier, place the head pillow so it does not force an acute neck angle. For example, place just the back half of the head on the pillow, allowing the face to angle downward (fig.4-8). Also, most people have a tendency to sway the lower back when lying face down. Placing a small pillow under the abdomen reduces the sway (fig.4-9). Before lying on your stomach, it pays to lengthen your spine by digging your elbows into the bed as you lay your torso down (fig.4-10). Young children sometimes sleep face down in a crouched position (fig.4-11).

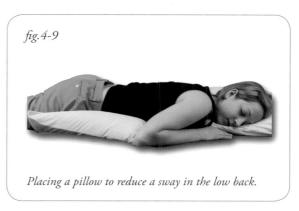

Placing a pillow to reduce a sway in the low back.

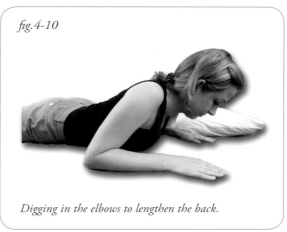

Digging in the elbows to lengthen the back.

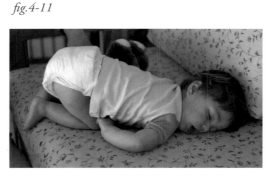

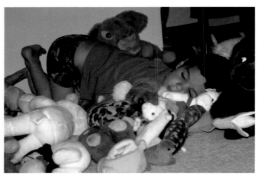

Young children have sufficient flexibility to sleep comfortably on their stomachs. They sometimes use a novel way to keep their backs well aligned.

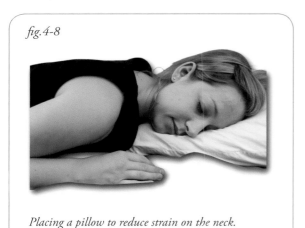

Placing a pillow to reduce strain on the neck.

WHAT TO DO WITH YOUR LEGS

Many people who sleep on their sides find it comfortable to straighten their lower leg, bend their upper knee, and twist their spine to place the upper knee on the bed (fig.4-12). If you have compressed discs, a twist in the spine can be dangerous. The position can be made healthy by lengthening the spine adequately before introducing the twist, and placing a pillow beneath the bent knee (fig.4-13).

fig.4-13

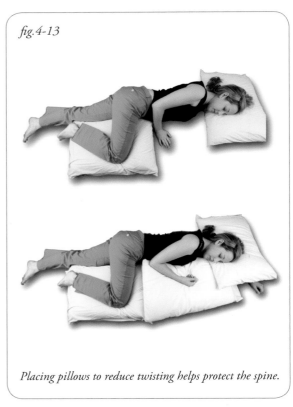

fig.4-12

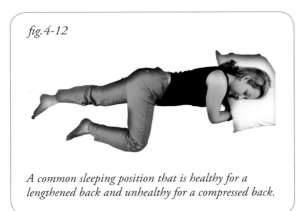

A common sleeping position that is healthy for a lengthened back and unhealthy for a compressed back.

Placing pillows to reduce twisting helps protect the spine.

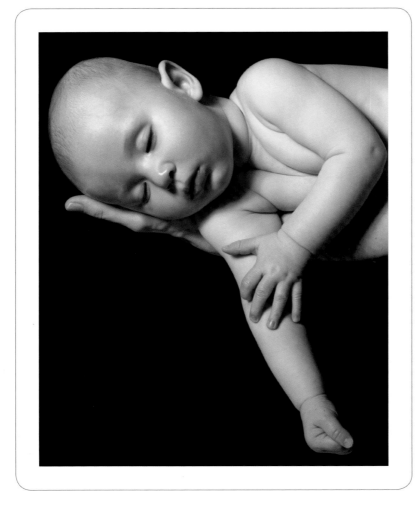

RECAP

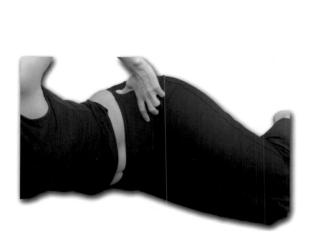

a. Tip pelvis forward, position buttocks well back, and bend knees to about 120° in a "zig-zag" fashion

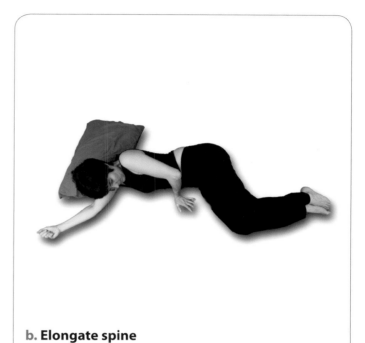

b. Elongate spine

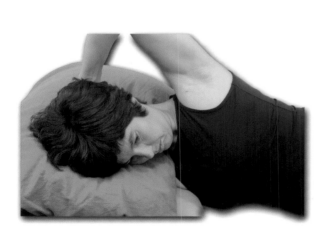

c. Lengthen neck onto pillow

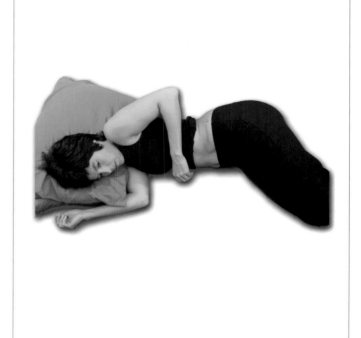

d. Perform shoulder roll with upper shoulder

5

USING YOUR INNER CORSET

Using your muscles to protect and lengthen your spine

My son reaches up for a toy. Notice that his abdominal muscles are engaged to help him elongate his torso to better reach the toy, his back is not swayed, and his head turns so that his eyes remain on a plane perpendicular to his body.

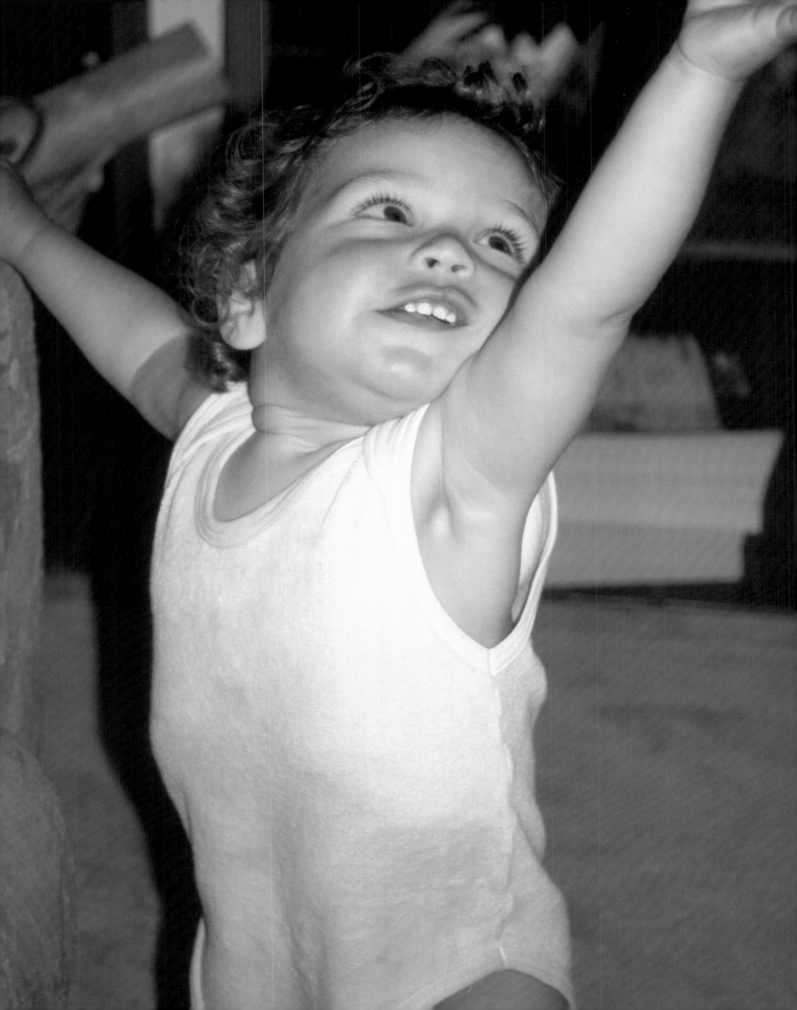

In the lessons so far, you have learned several effective ways to lengthen and protect your spine:

- Using an external object like a back rest or bed to put your spine in traction
- Positioning your pelvis so the vertebrae stack above it without tightening and shortening the surrounding muscles
- Breathing with the muscles around the spine relaxed, to further lengthen the spine with each inhalation

In this lesson you will learn a more powerful technique that gives you added length, is available to you at all times, and provides strong support to protect your elongated spine. The technique involves contracting certain muscles in your abdomen and back to make an "inner corset." This contraction causes the torso to become narrower and taller, thus lengthening the spine (fig.5-1).

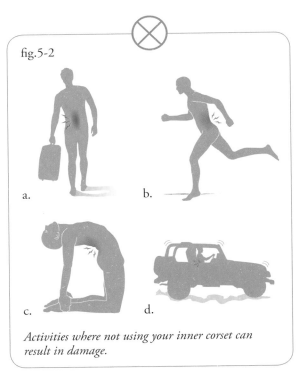

fig.5-2

a.   b.

c.   d.

Activities where not using your inner corset can result in damage.

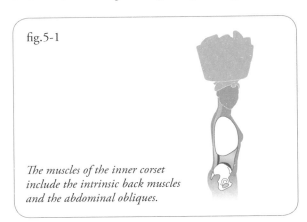

fig.5-1

The muscles of the inner corset include the intrinsic back muscles and the abdominal obliques.

The inner corset is important in situations where your discs may be challenged, such as:
- Carrying a heavy back pack, suit-case, or other object (fig.5-2a)
- Running, jogging, or engaging in other high-impact aerobic activities (fig.5-2b)
- Playing almost any sport – tennis, volleyball, basketball, or even swimming
- Performing Yoga poses that involve twists, side-bends, or backbends (fig.5-2c)
- Dancing in a way that involves impact, spinal twisting, or bending
- Riding on a bumpy road in a vehicle with poor shock absorbers, riding a mountain bike, or sailing in rough seas (fig.5-2d)

When an African or Indian village woman carries a heavy weight on her head (fig.5-3), she is not

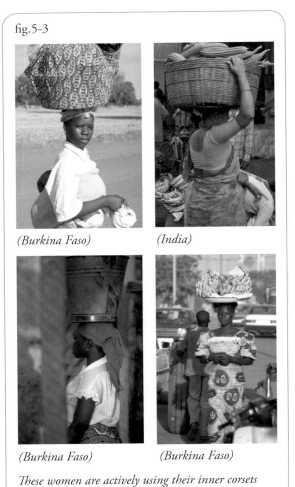

fig.5-3

(Burkina Faso)   *(India)*

(Burkina Faso)   *(Burkina Faso)*

These women are actively using their inner corsets to elongate and protect their spines as they carry substantial weights on their heads.

passive under that weight, which would cause her discs to compress. Rather, she actively engages her inner corset; her torso becomes more slender and her spine becomes longer. In this way she protects her discs from the weight she carries. Periodically, when carrying a burden for a long time, she may lift the burden above her head with outstretched arms (fig.5-4). This action stretches her back muscles and re-engages her inner corset.

Medical literature documents that in certain populations, such as the Bhil tribe of Central India, the discs of a 50-year-old look very similar to those of a 20-year-old (fig.5-5).[29] The proper and frequent use of the inner corset muscles is perhaps why these populations experience virtually no disc degeneration as they age. In our culture, on the other hand, it is considered normal to have significant disc degeneration by age 50. By using our muscles to protect our discs as the Bhils do, we can avoid the deterioration and damage that we have erroneously come to accept as normal.

In the Gokhale Method[SM], as in conventional approaches, there is an emphasis on using and strengthening the abdominal muscles. In our culture, when people use their abdominal

fig.5-4

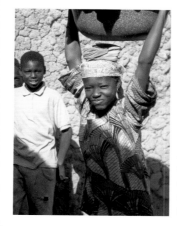

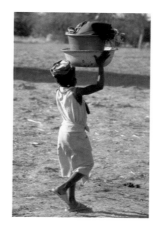

It is common among people who carry weights on their heads to stretch their back muscles and re-engage their inner corsets periodically.

Placing laundry basket on head (Burkina Faso)

fig.5-5

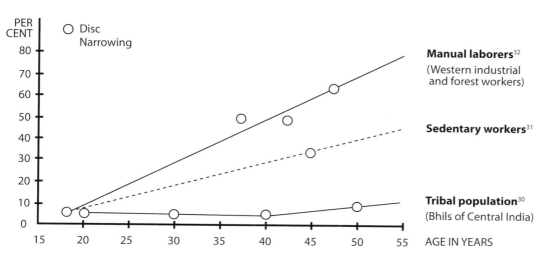

This graph [30] shows a large difference in disc narrowing with age in three different populations. There is very little disc narrowing in the Bhil tribal people of Central India,[29] more disc narrowing among Western sedentary workers,[30] and high levels of disc narrowing among Western industrial and forestry workers.[31]

musculature, they tend to use all their abdominals at once, tucking their pelvis and hunching their shoulders in the process (fig.5-6a). The result can be unhealthy posture (fig.5-6b).

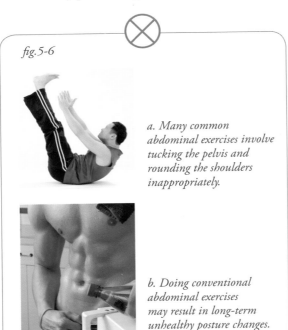

fig.5-6

a. Many common abdominal exercises involve tucking the pelvis and rounding the shoulders inappropriately.

b. Doing conventional abdominal exercises may result in long-term unhealthy posture changes.

In this lesson you will learn to isolate the abdominal *oblique* and *transversus* muscles from the *rectus abdominis* muscles so that you can lengthen and support your spine without distorting it. Learning this can be challenging, especially for some highly trained athletes who must overcome firmly ingrained habits to isolate the action of the different abdominal muscles.

The best way to strengthen and maintain these muscles is to use them in the course of daily activities. When you are first learning to use your abdominals in this new way, try to exercise your inner corset up to 20 times a day for a minute each time. This will help you establish the new pattern and reach a threshold level of muscle strength. It will also give your long back (*erector spinae*) muscles a periodic stretch and your discs a periodic decompression.

When you have integrated this new pattern into your daily life, you will find that many activities traditionally considered harmful for the back are actually healthy challenges for the muscles of your inner corset.

BENEFITS

- Stretches your spine more reliably and with a stronger action than any other technique

- Stabilizes your spine in case of injury

- Protects your spine in actions that involve compression, impact, or distortion

- Provides a stable platform enhancing the power of arm and leg actions

- Improves the tone and appearance of your torso

Until I met Esther Gokhale, I had lost hope in finding relief for my constant pain caused by a severe, multi-level back injury. I had spent years working with numerous physicians and physical therapists, received a number of cortisone injections, tried virtually every available prescription anti-inflammatory medication, and endured painful diagnostic and therapeutic procedures to curb significant pain and avoid surgery. I was convinced I had explored every treatment option, but I hadn't. Upon receiving independent endorsements of Esther's technique from trusted friends, I decided to see her for pain relief.

Initially I resented her advice to revisit the way I positioned and moved my body. I felt betrayed because I had faithfully followed my prescribed physical therapy and home exercise regime. Nevertheless, I was taught and slowly relearned how to sit, stand, walk, and even lie down.

I found and strengthened areas I didn't even know needed attention. With Esther's guidance, I worked out in new ways. Friends started telling me I looked great. Thank you, Esther, for relief from pain and a new awareness of my body.

Patti Fry
Menlo Park, CA

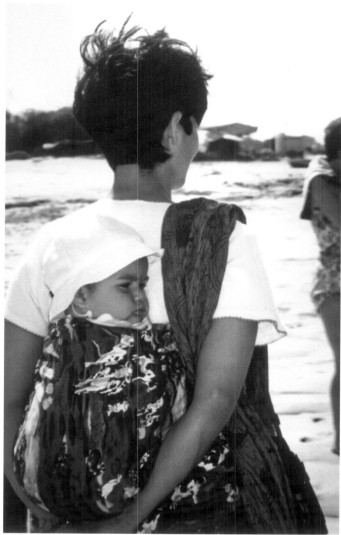

Carrying baby on back African-style

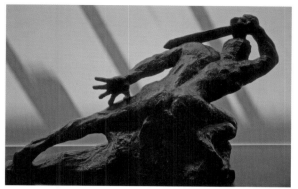

Gladiator sculpture (19th century, France)

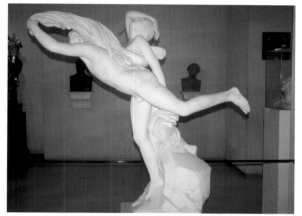

Yoga-like fantasy pose (19th century, France)

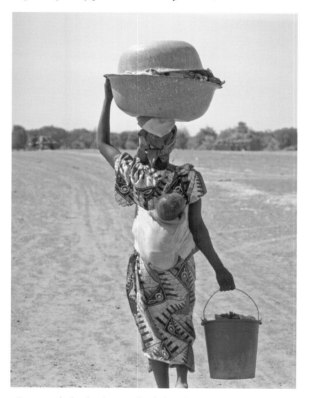

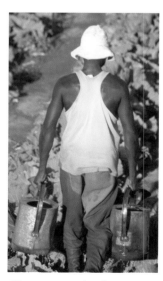

Watering crops (Burkina Faso)

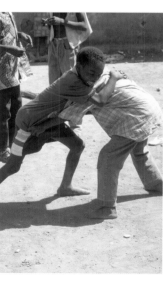

Wrestling game (Burkina Faso)

Carrying baby, bucket, and tub (Burkina Faso)

EQUIPMENT

You will need the following:
• *A full-length mirror*
• *A chair with a firm seat*
• *A wedge*

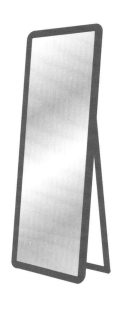

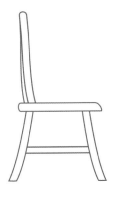

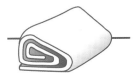

1 STACKSIT IN PROFILE TO THE MIRROR

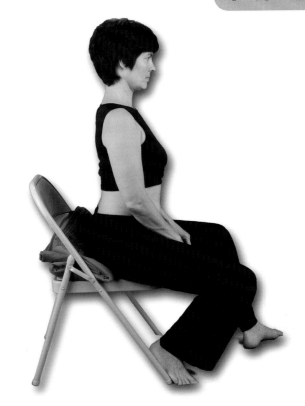

It is important to start with a healthy passive sitting position before engaging your inner corset.

2 PLACE THE FINGERTIPS OF YOUR LEFT HAND SO THEY CAN MONITOR YOUR SPINAL GROOVE

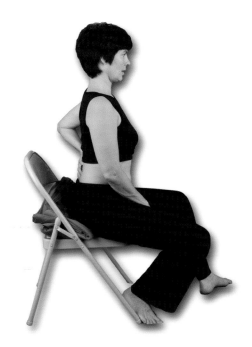

Use a light touch to check the entire low back. Ideally, you will have an even groove (see pages 77 and 133).

3 WITH YOUR RIGHT HAND, REACH UPWARD AND A LITTLE FORWARD, AS THOUGH YOU WERE REACHING FOR THE TOP OF A HIGH CABINET

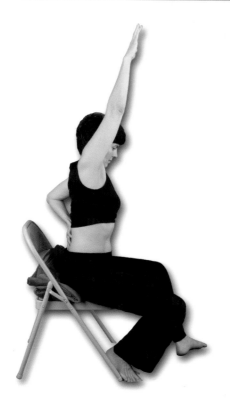

Try to find the direction of stretch that gives you length in your back rather than your front. Using feedback from your fingertips, maintain your spinal groove. It may help to imagine you are reaching up and over a bar at chest height.

4 REACH UP WITH YOUR LEFT HAND. KEEP YOUR ARMS PARALLEL AND STRETCH UPWARD AS FAR AS YOU CAN

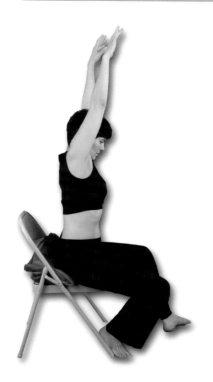

Become aware of the muscles in your abdomen. Engage them so that your abdomen feels sleeker than usual. The outline of your ribcage may become prominent, like that of a greyhound.

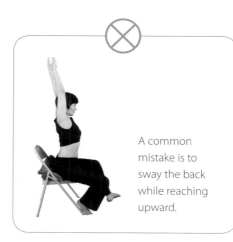

A common mistake is to sway the back while reaching upward.

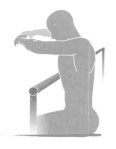

Imagine reaching up and over a bar at chest height to help engage the inner corset muscles correctly.

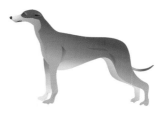

The lean abdominal area of a greyhound provides a useful image to help you engage your inner corset.

EXAMPLE OF ENGAGING THE INNER CORSET WHILE REACHING UP

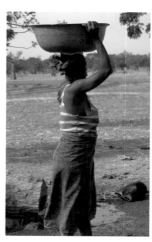

(Burkina Faso)

USING THE INNER CORSET TO PROTECT SPINAL STRUCTURES

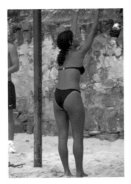

Preparing to pull up (Brazil)

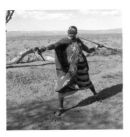

Hunting with a spear (Tanzania)

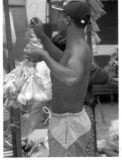

Hanging wares in stall (Brazil)

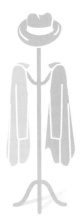

A coat rack provides a useful image to help you maintain a stable torso while relaxing your shoulders and arms.

5 SLOWLY LOWER YOUR ARMS AND RELAX YOUR SHOULDERS

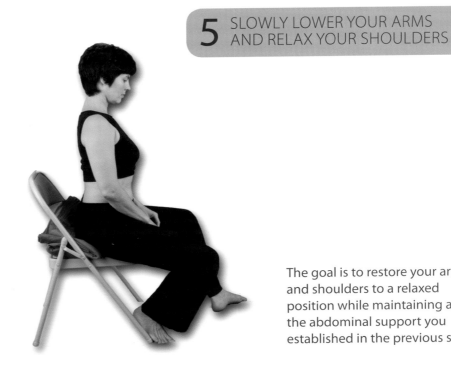

The goal is to restore your arms and shoulders to a relaxed position while maintaining all the abdominal support you established in the previous step.

6 REPEAT STEPS 2-5 WHILE STANDING

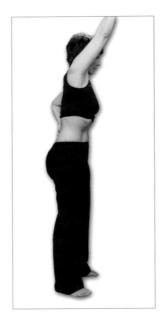
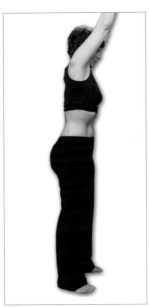
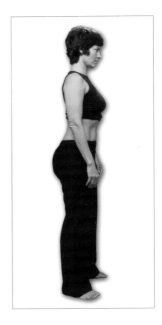

As before, be careful to lengthen rather than arch or round the back. It is difficult to isolate the inner abdominal muscles. You may find, as many beginners do, that when you relax your arms and shoulders, your abdominal muscles relax too. If so, start again and proceed with care. Imagine that you are a coat rack: The spine is the sturdy, tall central support and the shoulder girdle is a coat hanging from it.

7 PRACTICE MAINTAINING THIS INNER CORSET AS YOU MOVE

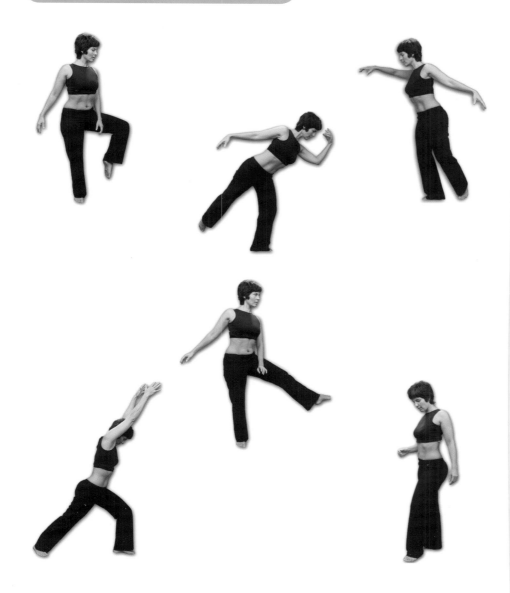

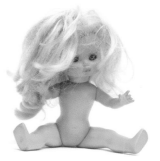

Imagine you are a marionette or doll with a stable torso and freely-moving limbs.

You may feel a bit like a marionette; the torso is relatively still and stable, while the limbs are available for movement.

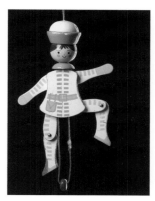

EXAMPLE OF MOVING THE LIMBS WHILE KEEPING THE TORSO TALL AND STABLE

8 PRACTICE RELAXING AND ENGAGING THE INNER CORSET MUSCLES REPEATEDLY

With time and practice you will no longer need to use your arms to find this action. Your body will learn to do it very quickly when needed.

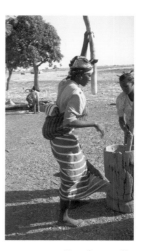

Grinding millet (Burkina Faso)

EXAMPLES OF ENGAGING
THE INNER CORSET:

ENJOYING
YOUTHFUL
ACTIVITIES
(Brazil)

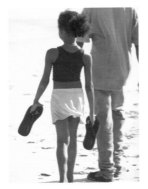

PERFORMING
MANUAL LABOR
(Brazil)

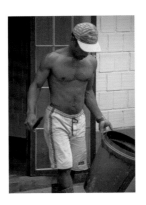

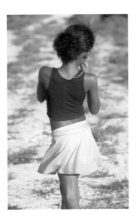 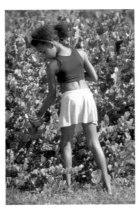

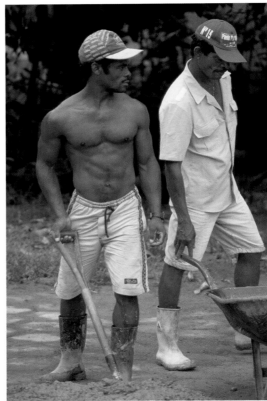

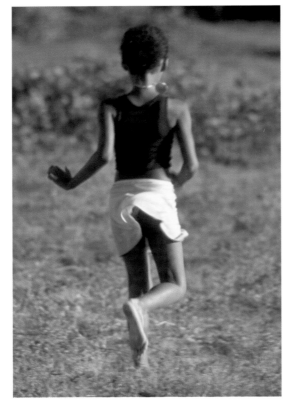

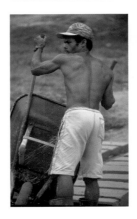 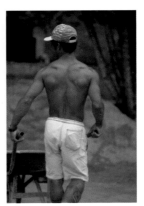

"PLAYING" CAPOEIRA,
A CHALLENGING MARTIAL ART
(Brazil)

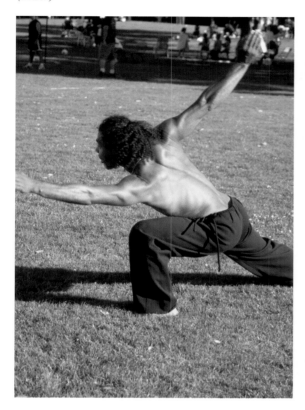

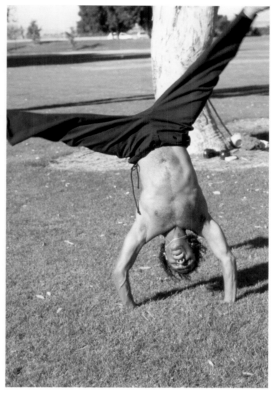

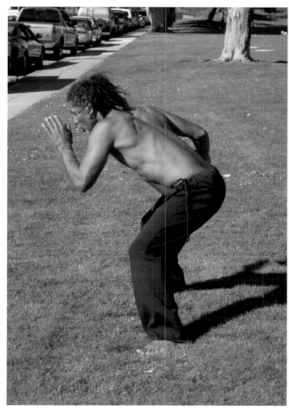

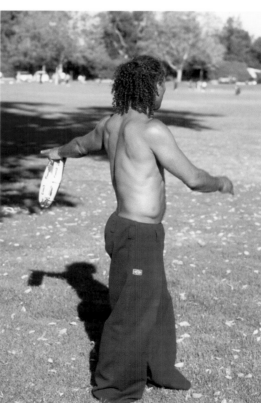

INDICATIONS OF IMPROVEMENT

Using the inner corset can be difficult to learn because your abdominal muscles may not be strong, you may not be used to isolating them, and the long muscles of your back (*erector spinae*) may resist the action. With practice, as your inner corset muscles get stronger, and as your long back muscles become more limber, the pattern will be easier to maintain. You will also no longer need the raised arm action to engage the inner corset.

Once you start using your abdominal muscles during your daily activities, they become toned very quickly. After some time, you may be able to see their contours on your abdomen even when you are not flexing your muscles (fig.5-7).

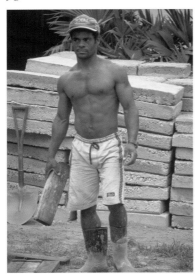

fig.5-7

The contours of this worker's abdominal muscles are apparent even when he is relaxed (Brazil).

TROUBLESHOOTING

SWAYING THE LOW BACK

This is the most common mistake when learning to elongate your torso (see page 117). Monitoring your spinal groove with one hand as you start to lengthen your back will help you detect the sway and prevent it from happening. If your abdominal muscles need strengthening, you will find suitable exercises in Appendix 1. I recommend doing those exercises regularly until your abdominal muscles reach a threshold level of strength.

DIFFICULTY BREATHING

If you are accustomed to breathing with your abdomen and not your chest, you may find it difficult to inhale deeply while engaging your inner corset. As part of your inner corset, your abdominal muscles are contracted and resist abdominal expansion during inhalation. But the muscles between your ribs (*intercostals*) may be stiff from a lack of action in the past, and resist chest expansion during inhalation. You will therefore be hampered in your ability to inhale easily. By forcing a few deep inhalations, you stretch your intercostal muscles, making subsequent inhalations easier. Soon you will be able to breathe deeply and easily while engaging your inner corset.

FURTHER INFORMATION

LENGTHENING BY CONTRACTING

You might ask how you can lengthen your spine by contracting your muscles. The answer is two-fold.

First, contracting the abdominal muscles causes the abdomen to become narrower. Since the abdomen has a fixed volume, it must become taller, changing its shape from a short, squat cylinder to a tall, thin cylinder (fig.5-8). This action elongates the spine, easing the vertebrae apart and decompressing the discs. The low back feels braced, as though you were wearing the support belt commonly used by workers who carry heavy burdens. You use an inner corset made of your own muscles.

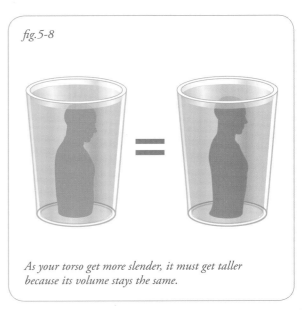

fig.5-8

As your torso get more slender, it must get taller because its volume stays the same.

Second, certain muscles, because of their geometry, cause the spine to lengthen as they contract. For example, the *longus colli* muscles are located in front of the cervical spine. When these muscles contract, they force the cervical curve to straighten, thus lengthening the cervical spine (fig.5-9).

The deepest muscles of the back (*rotatores*) have a more complex geometry. When used unilaterally (that is, on just one side of the spine), the rotatores muscles cause the spine to rotate. When used bilaterally, these muscles cause the spine to elongate. It is difficult to envision how this works but we know from electro-myelographic studies that these muscles are involved in lengthening the spine.

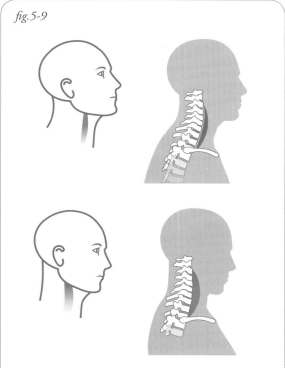

fig.5-9

The longus colli muscles attach to the front (anterior) part of the neck (cervical) spine. When they contract, they cause the neck to straighten and, therefore, lengthen.

JUMPING

Although using your inner corset may seem like a contrived action, you automatically use it whenever your spine is subject to extreme stress. For example, when you jump down from a significant height, you instinctively tighten your inner corset to protect your spine (fig.5-10).

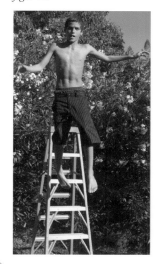

fig.5-10

The inner corset muscles automatically contract in high stress situations like jumping.

In situations of moderate stress, however, most people do not have the instinct to use the same protective mechanism. Failure to do so can lead to cumulative damage of spinal structures, damage that we have come to consider a normal part of aging in our culture. By learning to use the inner corset in these situations, you will protect your back from this damage. At the same time, you will be exercising your abdominal muscles.

REACHING ABOVE YOUR HEAD

A conventional guideline for patients with low back pain is to avoid reaching above the head, as when reaching for a glass on a high shelf or placing luggage in an overhead compartment. If done carelessly, this is indeed a dangerous maneuver. However, by anchoring the rib cage (see Appendix 1) and engaging the inner corset, you can reach up more safely with the side benefit of strengthening the abdominal muscles (fig.5-11).

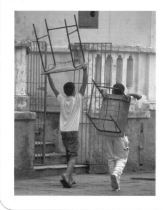

fig.5-11

Reaching upwards can be a helpful way to engage the inner corset muscles.

PROTECTING YOUR NECK

Just as the inner corset protects the vulnerable lumbar discs, engaging the *longus colli* muscles protects the fragile cervical discs. People in traditional cultures do this when they carry significant weight on their heads. To learn this action, place a soft, light weight, such as a folded towel, on the crown of your head (fig.6-13a on page144). A common mistake is to place the weight too far forward on your head, causing the chin to rise and the neck to compress (fig.6-13c). Imagine this weight is heavy and actively push up against it (fig.6-13b). Be moderate in this pushing action and only sustain the push for a few seconds.

USING AN EXTERNAL CORSET

Many people assume that corsets are uncomfortable and unhealthy. In fact, some corsets, such as those used in the 18th century, protected and supported the back (fig.5-12). It is true that in Victorian times, some corsets became extreme and unhealthy (fig.5-13). Yet a moderate corset remains a healthy device; weight lifters regularly wear back support belts, as do workers who carry heavy objects (fig.5-14). The medical profession also prescribes corsets for back pain patients to correct distortions or protect damaged tissues. Simple versions of these are available at medical supply stores and can be useful if you are injured.

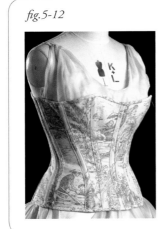

fig.5-12

This early corset is moderate and healthful.

With inner or external corsets, some people fear loss of flexibility and spinal health. Interestingly, among the Dinkas of Southern Sudan, young people wear corsets with rigid metal ribbing to show their status (fig.5-15). These corsets are worn day and night for years. The only way to remove a Dinka corset is to cut it, which is done only when a larger size is needed. The corsets permit no appreciable flexion, extension, lateral bending, or twist in the spine. The excellent physique of the Dinka is testimony to how little spinal movement is truly needed to preserve good musculo-skeletal health.

fig.5-13

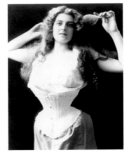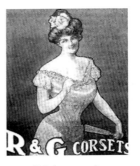

Some corsets in the Victorian era (19th century) became extreme and compromised health.

fig.5-14

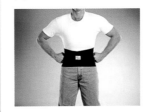

Modern back belts provide support for performing heavy manual labor or in case of injury.

fig.5-15

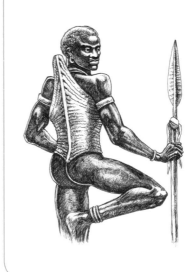

A Dinka corset from Sudan. These are worn day and night for years. Note that the L5-S1 area is allowed to assume its normal curvature.

Note that the Dinka corset stops at the level of the L5-S1 disc. It is interesting to contrast the Dinka corset with some of the more extensive modern medical corsets and devices. In my clinical experience, most patients, if they need a corset at all, do best with a corset that leaves the pelvis free to settle in an anteverted position. Unfortunately, many of the available medical devices, such as the TLSO body cast (fig.5-16), not only fix the pelvis, but fix it in a retroverted position. The TLSO, according to medical literature, has failed to demonstrate any substantial positive outcome.

An interesting case study from my practice involves K, who came into my care at age 13. She suffered from *kyphoscoliosis*, a condition in which her spine had excessive curves, both side-to-side and front-to-back. Her father, a physician, had been proactive in arranging care for his daughter. However, after seven months of physical therapy and two custom TLSO body casts supposed to be worn 20 hours a day for two years proved unsuccessful, doctors recommended surgery. The family was not keen on this route. I taught K how to sit, lie, stand, bend, and walk in the ways described in this book. Re-establishing pelvic anteversion and learning to hip-hinge were particularly important elements in her training. The immediate feedback in comfort and improved appearance motivated her strongly. Within two months, her outlook was radically different (fig.5-17). There was no further talk of surgery, body casts, physical therapy, or any other intervention. K is now in college and continues to strike people as a particularly good-looking and poised young lady.

fig.5-16

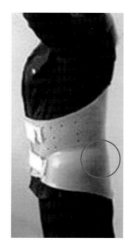

An example of a TLSO, a body cast used for children with scoliosis. Notice the flattening effect on the L5-S1 area.

fig.5-17

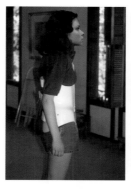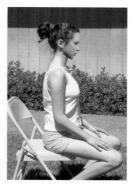
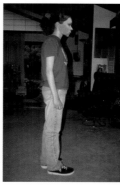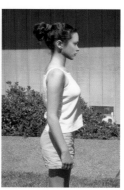
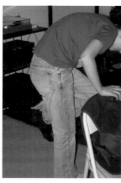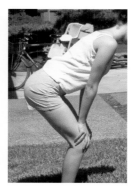
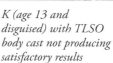

K (age 13 and disguised) with TLSO body cast not producing satisfactory results

K after 3 months of training with much-improved appearance and outlook (note the slight sway in the second photograph that she subsequently corrected).

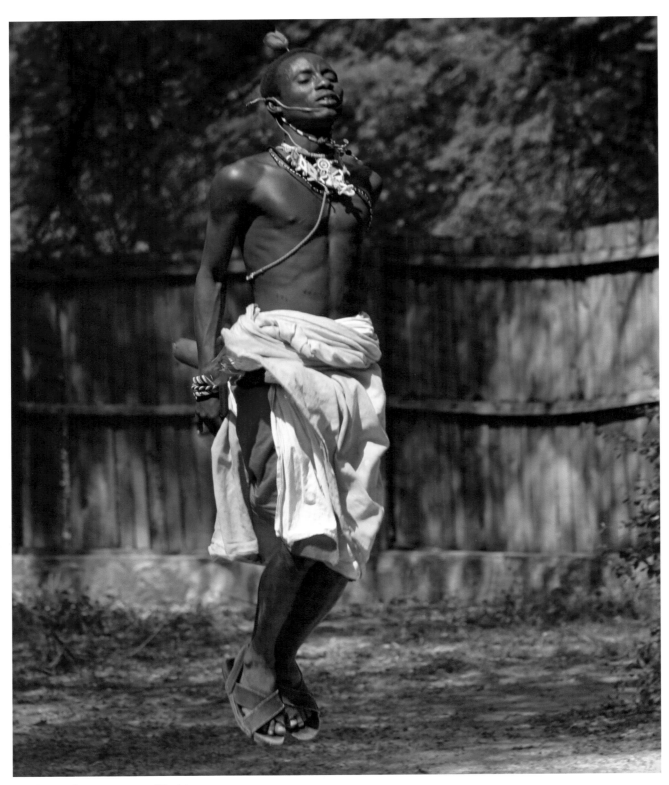

Samburu tribesman jumping (Kenya)

RECAP

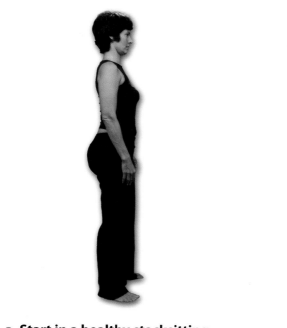

a. Start in a healthy stacksitting or standing position.

b. Monitor groove in back and reach high with one arm

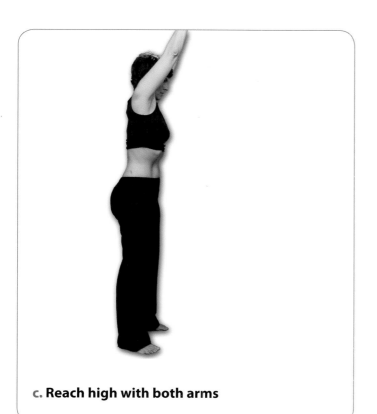

c. Reach high with both arms

d. Lower arms while maintaining inner corset

6

TALLSTANDING

Stacking your bones

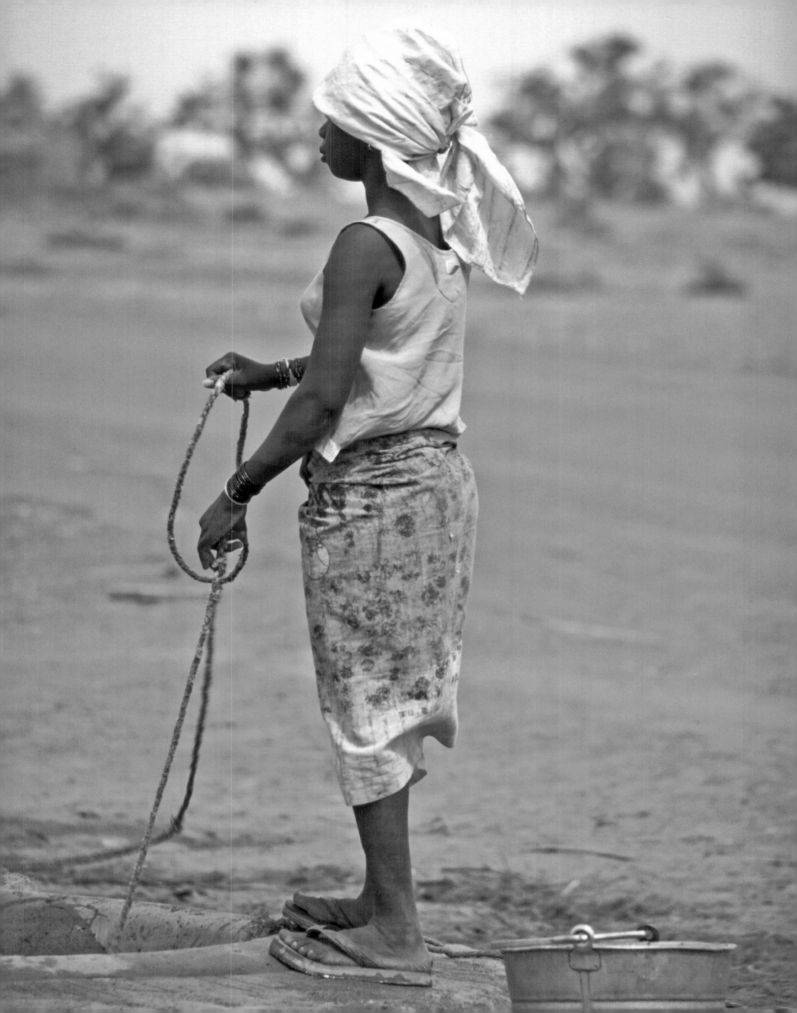

Many people are uncomfortable standing for long periods of time. If they go to a museum, their backs hurt; if they go to a party, their feet hurt. Yet many others stand comfortably all day to earn their living. A few, like the Inuit seal-hunters, stand without moving at all for long periods.

By learning how to tallstand, you will be able to stand for long periods without feeling fidgety or uncomfortable. Just as with healthy sitting, healthy standing requires tipping the pelvis forward and stacking the vertebrae. The hips align over the heels, which carry most of the body weight, and the knees and groin area remain soft (fig.6-1). The position facilitates healthy blood flow to and from the legs. Standing becomes a comfortable, even restful, position.

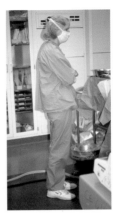
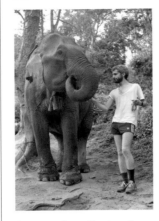

fig.6-2

Poor standing often involves a tucked pelvis that is thrust forward, impinging the femoral arteries, veins, and nerves.

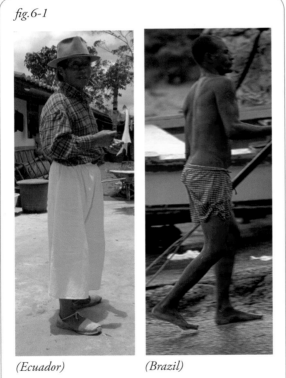

fig.6-1

(Ecuador)   (Brazil)

Healthy erect posture involves an anteverted pelvis and well-stacked vertebrae and leg bones.

Thrusting the hips forward is usually accompanied by excessive curvature in the spine, which strains the vertebrae, and places inappropriate stresses on hip joints (fig.6-3). It displaces the weight forward onto the delicate joints in the front of the foot, distorting the foot from its natural arched shape, and contributing to problems like bunions, plantar fasciitis, and arthritis of the foot (fig.6-4). The stance also creates a tendency to lock the knees, which strains the injury-prone knee ligaments and predisposes people to arthritis of the knee (fig.6-5).

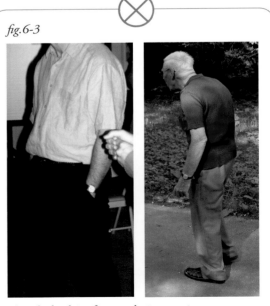

fig.6-3

A tucked pelvis often results in excessive curvature throughout the spine.

People who stand poorly often tuck their pelvis and park their hips forward, impinging the femoral artery and vein, and reducing blood flow to and from the legs (fig.6-2). Reduced blood flow slows the repair of any leg injuries and contributes to such problems as cold feet, Raynaud's syndrome, and varicose veins.

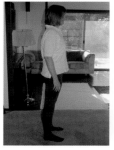
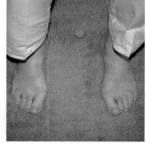

fig.6-4

A pelvis thrust forward displaces body weight forward, putting excessive pressure on the delicate structures in the front of the foot.

Excessive pressure on the front of the foot may result in bunions and other pathologies.

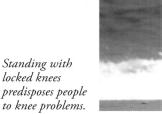
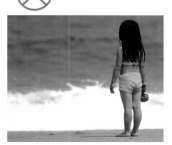

fig.6-5

Standing with locked knees predisposes people to knee problems.

Another common pattern of standing incorrectly is to sway the low back in an effort to "stand up straight" (fig.6-6). This strains the low back muscles and over time causes them to adapt to a shorter baseline length. Strained low back muscles cause compression in the low back (*lumbar*) discs and poor circulation in the low back in general.

fig.6-6

The directive to "stand up straight" often results in a swayed low back.

The secret to standing comfortably is a healthy vertical stacking of the body's weight-bearing bones coupled with healthy foot and leg alignment (fig.6-7, 6-8). Stacking provides a necessary and healthy stress for the bones, helping to prevent osteoporosis. Stacking also allows the muscles around the joints to relax. The bones get the stress they need, and the muscles are relieved of stress they *don't* need. Because the muscles can relax, they allow good blood circulation.

fig.6-7

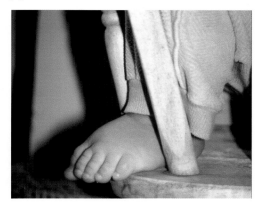

Healthy foot and leg alignment is an important part of healthy standing.

BENEFITS

- Prevents wear and tear on the feet, knees, and hips

- Reduces back pain from tight back muscles or compressed discs

- Enables standing for long periods without fatigue, pain, or damage

- Introduces healthy stress to the weight-bearing bones and helps to prevent osteoporosis

- Improves blood circulation in the legs and feet

fig.6-8

PELVIS TIPPED

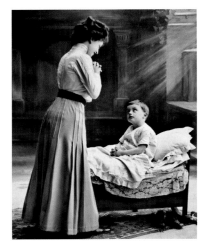

(USA)

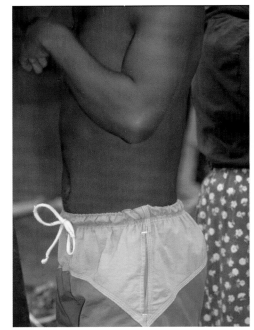

(Brazil)

LOW BACK STRAIGHT

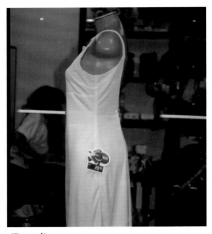

(Brazil)

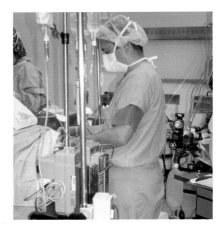

(USA)

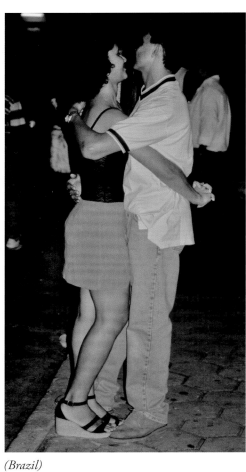

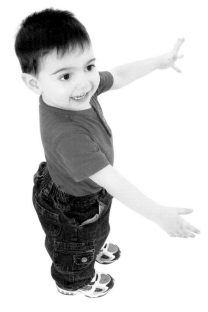

(Cambodia)   *(Brazil)*   *(USA)*

fig.6-8 (continued)

EVEN SPINAL GROOVE

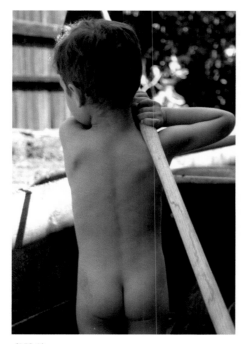

(USA)

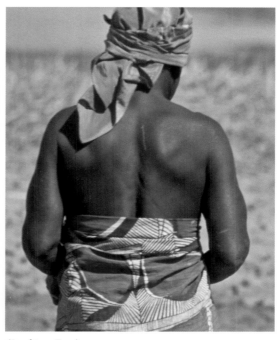

(Burkina Faso)

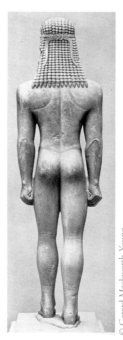

(Greece)

© Gerard Mackworth-Young

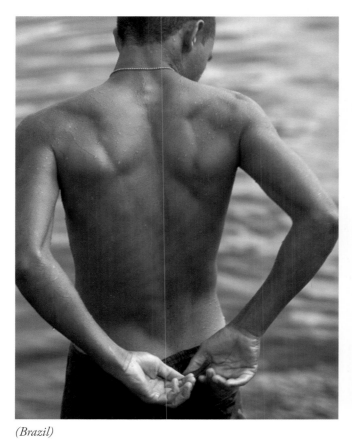

(Brazil)

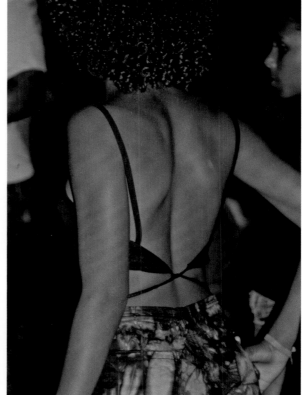

(Brazil)

EQUIPMENT

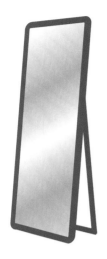

You will need a full-length mirror.

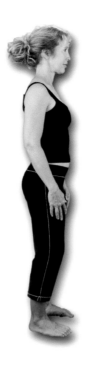

1 STAND ON A FIRM FLOOR WITH YOUR FEET HIP-WIDTH APART AND TURNED OUT 10°-15°

Because your feet are your foundation when you stand, it is important that they be arranged well. You will "shape" them in the next few steps.

2 RELEASE THE WEIGHT ON YOUR RIGHT FOOT. FIX THE TOES AND BALL OF THE FOOT ON THE FLOOR, AND RAISE THE HEEL SLIGHTLY

Leave your foot muscles relaxed as you do this.

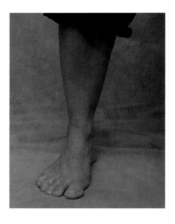
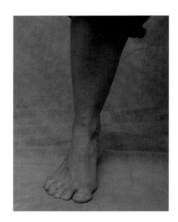

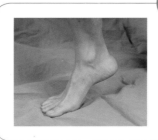

A common mistake is to raise the heel too high. This causes tension in the foot that prevents reshaping.

3 PIVOT THE HEEL INWARD BEFORE PLANTING IT FIRMLY ON THE FLOOR

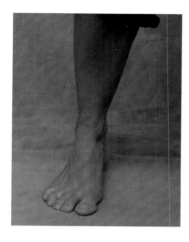

Note that this action emphasizes the inner arch of your foot, creating a "kidney-bean" shape. Also note that your legs will turn outwards ("externally rotate") in this step. In fact, focusing on externally rotating your knees can help you create a kidney-bean shape in your foot.

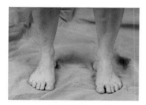
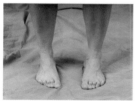

A common mistake is to pivot the front of the foot inward rather than the heel. This easily results in a "pigeon-toed" stance.

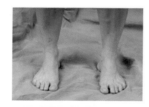
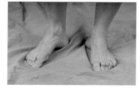

Another common mistake is to let the ball of the foot pivot outward as the heel moves inward. This simply increases the splay of the foot rather than changing its shape.

4 IF NECESSARY, USE YOUR HANDS TO GUIDE THE MOVEMENT

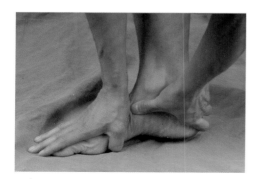

Steady the front of the foot with one hand. Grasp the heel with the other hand, lift the heel from the floor, and firmly pivot it inward.

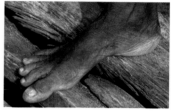

(India)

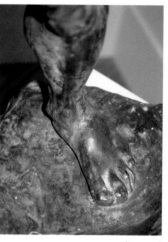

(France)

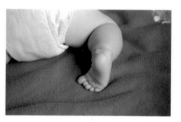

(USA)

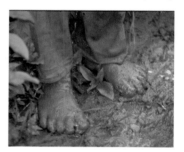

(Thailand)

Kidney-bean shaped feet are a function of strong tibialis anterior muscles (see Appendix 1 for exercises to strengthen this muscle).

EXAMPLES OF HEALTHY FOOT STRUCTURE FROM AROUND THE WORLD

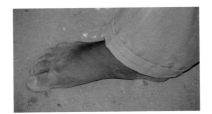

(Burkina Faso)

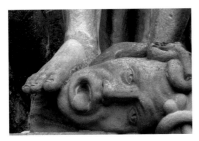

(Germany)

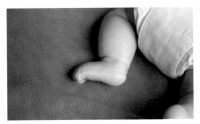

(USA)

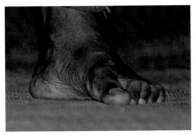

This Kathakali dancer from South India keeps his feet in the traditional, slightly exaggerated kidney-bean shape with the weight somewhat to the outside of the foot.

5 ROLL YOUR ANKLE SLIGHTLY INWARD

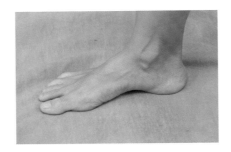

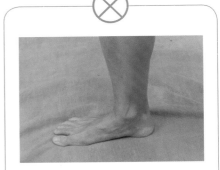

This subtle movement evens the weight between the inside and the outside of the foot.

A common mistake is to *pronate* the foot excessively. If you cannot prevent this, use an insole (see page 146).

6 SHRINK THE LENGTH OF YOUR FOOT

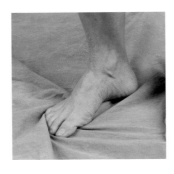

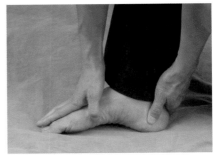

Engage the arch muscles to pull the front of the foot closer to the heel. If necessary, use your hands to assist you.

7 REPEAT STEPS 2 THROUGH 6 WITH THE LEFT FOOT

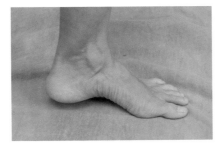

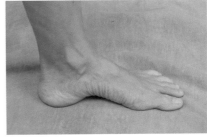

8 CHECK THAT YOUR KNEES AND LEGS ARE ROTATED SLIGHTLY OUTWARDS

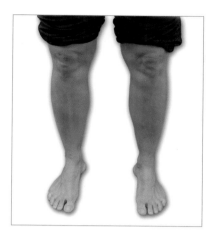

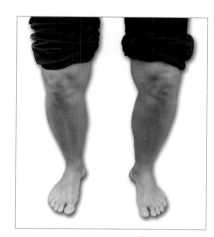

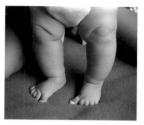

(USA)

Bend your knees a little and check that your knees and feet are aligned. Imagine that a line runs outward from your heel through the second or third toe. Your knee should point along this line.

A common mistake is to rotate the knees inward with the feet pointing outward.

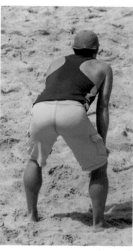

(Brazil)

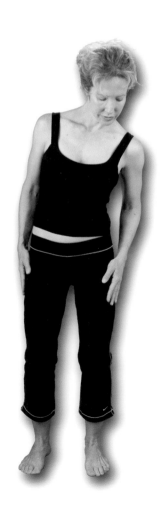

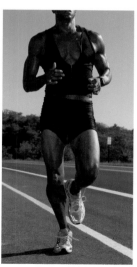

(USA)

You may have to shift your head over your knee to get an aerial view of the alignment.

EXTERNAL LEG ROTATION

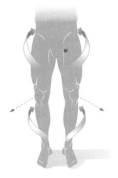

"Wrapping" your leg muscles outward externally rotates the entire leg, resulting in healthy alignment of the hip, knee, and ankle joints, and recreation of the inner arch of the foot. Two key muscles involved in this action are tibialis anterior (the shin splint muscle) and gluteus medius.

HEALTHY STANDING POSTURE FROM AROUND THE WORLD

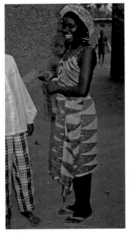

(Burkina Faso)

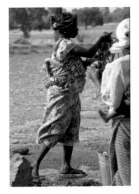

(Burkina Faso)

9 IF NECESSARY, "WRAP" YOUR LEG MUSCLES TO ROTATE YOUR LEGS OUTWARD

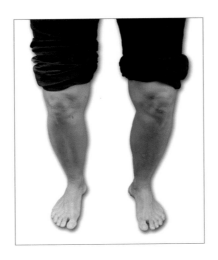

This action involves your gluteus and leg muscles.

10 REARRANGE YOUR WEIGHT TO FALL OVER YOUR HEELS

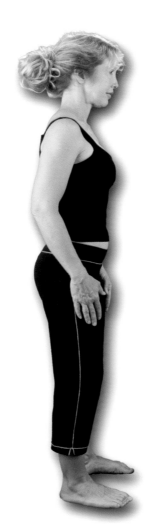

Stand in profile in front of a full-length mirror. Visualize an imaginary plumb line dropping from your hip joint to your feet. The plumb bob should fall close to the heel. If it does not, shift your hips back. Simultaneously bring your torso forward (bend at the hip, not the waist) so as not to topple backwards.

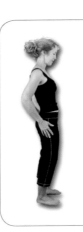

A common mistake is to place too much weight on the front of the feet. In this case, the plumb bob would fall significantly in front of your heel.

11 SOFTEN THE KNEES AND GROIN AREA

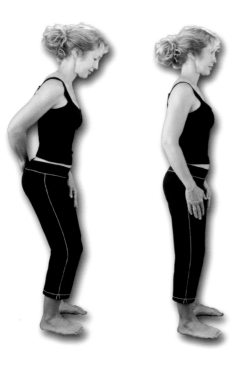

If you have trouble softening the groin area, sink downward, bending equally at the knees and hip joints in an accordion fashion. Note that now your torso is parallel to your lower legs, and your pelvis "nests" between your legs. Leaving the weight on the heels, slowly straighten just short of locking the knees or the groin.

At first you may feel that you are canted forward, but a glance in the mirror will reassure you.

12 CHECK THE GROIN CREASE FOR SOFTNESS

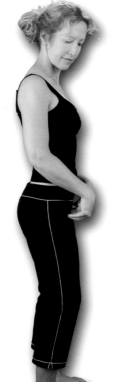

Place your fingers where the top of the legs hinge at the hip. If you have not locked your groin, you should feel some "give" in the soft tissue before feeling bone.

HEALTHY STANDING POSTURE FROM AROUND THE WORLD

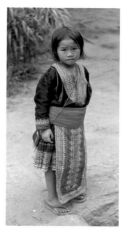

(Thailand)

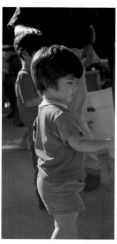

(USA)

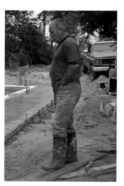

(USA)

ART PIECES SHOWING TALLSTANDING

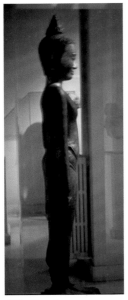

(Thailand)

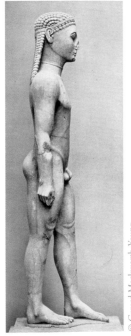

© Gerard Mackworth-Young

(Greece)

13 RELAX THE MUSCLES IN YOUR LOW BACK, ALLOWING THE RIBCAGE TO SETTLE INTO ITS BASELINE POSITION

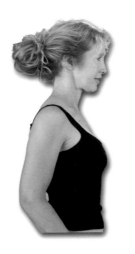

In this position, the bottom of the ribcage on your front is flush with the contour of the torso. If necessary, contract the abdominal oblique muscles to anchor the bottom of the ribcage.

To check that your low back muscles are relaxed, breathe deeply. If your low back is relaxed, it will lengthen as you inhale.

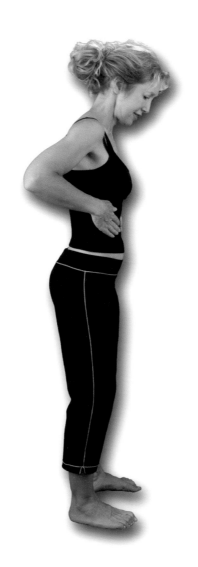

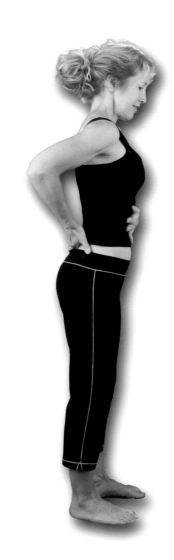

14 PERFORM A SLOW SHOULDER ROLL WITH EACH SHOULDER, SETTLING IT IN ITS DOWN-AND-BACK POSITION

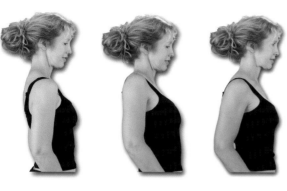

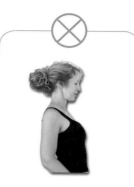

A common mistake is to sway the back when doing a shoulder roll.

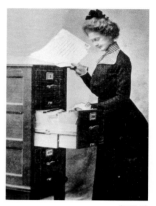

(USA)

Keep your rib anchor engaged. Be sure you don't unwittingly tighten and sway your low back as you settle your shoulders.

15 LENGTHEN YOUR NECK; CHECK FOR AND RELEASE ANY TENSION

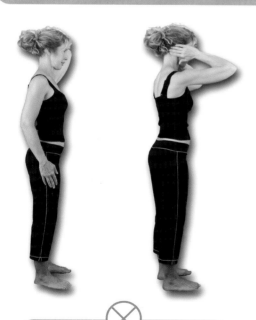

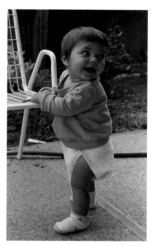

(USA)

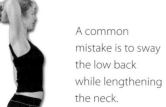

A common mistake is to sway the low back while lengthening the neck.

Your head should settle into its natural position with the chin angled slightly downward.

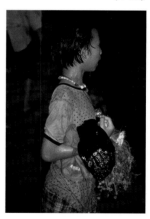

(Thailand)

INDICATIONS OF IMPROVEMENT

If you are used to standing with your hips thrust forward, your groin and knees locked, and your torso leaning backwards to maintain balance, you may feel like a chimpanzee in this new stance. Stand sideways to a mirror and look at your profile, especially from the shoulders down. This will reassure you that you are in fact vertically aligned. Give your brain some time to reset; soon the awkwardness will fade.

As you alter your stance, you will notice these specific changes in your feet:

- Each foot maintains a kidney-bean shape and has strong musculature.
- Each foot has well-developed inner, outer, and transverse arches.
- At rest, your feet naturally splay outward 10°-15°.

fig.6-8

(USA)

(Ireland)

(Burkina Faso)

As you change your stance you will notice the following features in your feet: kidney bean shape, pronounced arches, and a 10º-15º splay (eversion).

TROUBLESHOOTING

UNABLE TO CONTRACT THE FOOT ARCH MUSCLES

If you have difficulty attaining a kidney-bean shape in your feet, even when you use your hands, you may need someone's help (fig.6-9). You will soon be able to do it on your own. If you have considerable rigidity in your feet, consider using massage to help increase flexibility.

If you have difficulty shortening your foot, you may also want guidance from your own or someone else's hands. The goal is to engage the arch muscles while allowing the toes to remain relaxed. When learning this action, many people experience tension around the toes. Be patient; with time, you will isolate your arch muscles better, releasing the tension in your toes.

fig.6-9

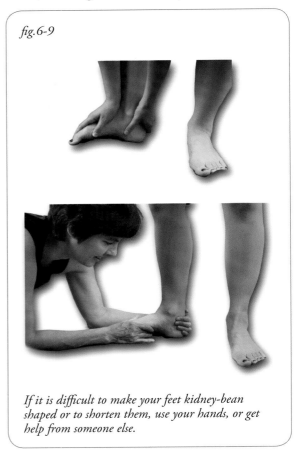

If it is difficult to make your feet kidney-bean shaped or to shorten them, use your hands, or get help from someone else.

DIFFICULTY SHIFTING WEIGHT ONTO HEELS

Here is a simple way to shift your weight onto your heels: Very slowly bend forward and then backward at the groin (fig.6-10). Try to use a minimum of muscular effort. Gradually decrease the amplitude of your forward and backward bends until you settle at a balance point. You will discover that your weight is now mainly on your heels.

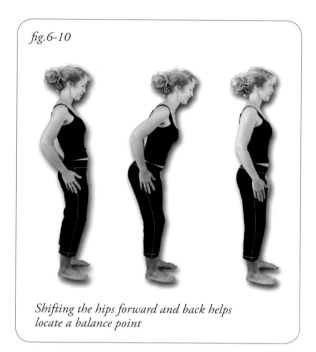

fig.6-10

Shifting the hips forward and back helps locate a balance point

If you still find it challenging to shift your weight to your heels, try placing a small superball (about 1/2" in diameter) under the transverse arch of each foot (fig.6-11). These will help you identify where your weight falls. If you carry your weight forward over the arches of your feet, the balls will feel very uncomfortable.

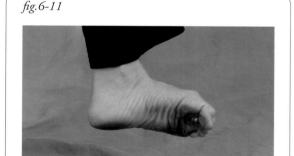

fig.6-11

Placing small superballs under the transverse arch of the foot behind your toes can train you to leave your weight on your heels. It can also help to strengthen your foot arch muscles.

PROBLEMS ALIGNING THE SHOULDERS

Sometimes it is helpful to use an aid for shoulder alignment. Have a friend gently tie your upper arms behind you. Use a long piece of cloth or small sheet and fold it several times to make a thick band. Then run it under your arms and tie the ends so that the shoulder blades are drawn close together behind you (fig.6-12). Make sure you are comfortable, that your circulation is not compromised, and that you are maintaining a neutral position in your back (do not allow your ribs to jut out in the front as your shoulders are drawn back). This puts your shoulders in better alignment than you can achieve on your own, and gives you one less body part to monitor.

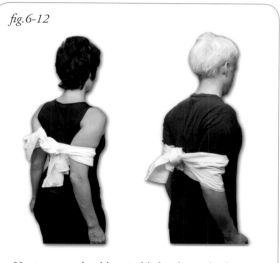

fig.6-12

Having your shoulders tied behind your back can help you experience good shoulder alignment without strain.

INABILITY TO SENSE YOUR VERTICAL AXIS

You may be unsure whether you have successfully learned to tallstand. If you want to sense your new vertical axis, place a light weight, such as a folded hand towel, on the crown of your head (fig.6-13). This will help you find a good alignment and make you aware of any habitual or excessive movements that pull you out of alignment.

To move even closer to your ideal vertical axis, you can push upward and engage the *longus colli* muscles (just in front of your cervical spine) (fig.6-13b). People who carry significant weight on their heads use this action to protect their spines (fig.6-14). You can also use this technique when learning to sit well and walk well (see

Lessons 3 and 8, respectively). Note that until your neck is well-aligned and your neck muscles strong, you should not try to place a heavy weight on your head.

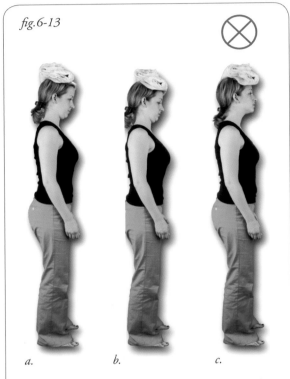

fig.6-13

a.   *b.*   *c.*

a) Placing a light weight (that will not hurt you if it falls) on the crown of your head can help you locate your vertical axis. b) Push up against the weight to engage your longus colli muscles. c) A common mistake is to carry the weight too far forward on your head.

fig.6-14

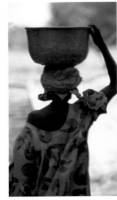
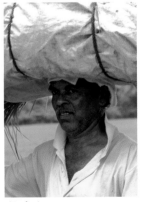

(Burkina Faso)   *(India)*

People who carry weight on their head push up against the weight using their neck (longus colli) muscles as well as their inner corset. In this way, they sustain no damage from the weight.

FURTHER INFORMATION

ARM POSITION

When standing for an extended period of time, people in traditional cultures usually rest their arms on some part of their bodies (fig.6-22 on page 148). In all the photographs, the shoulders retain a healthy alignment. This is even true when the arms are folded across the front. (Beginners should avoid this position because it can easily lead to hunched shoulders.)

Notice that when the arms do hang by the side of the body (fig.6-15), they hang to the back of the torso and the thumbs face forward or, when carrying, are externally rotated (fig.6-16).

fig.6-15

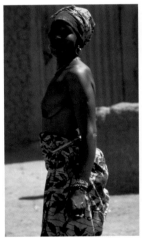
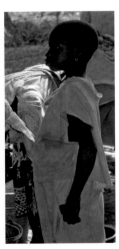

(Burkina Faso)   *(Burkina Faso)*

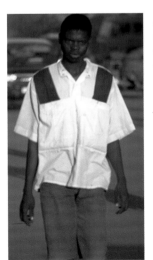

In traditional cultures, when the arms hang at the sides, they align well back along the torso with the thumbs facing forward.

(Burkina Faso)

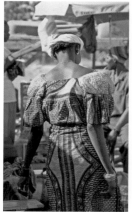
(Burkina Faso)

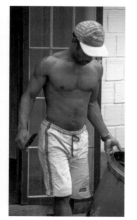
(Brazil)

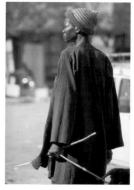
(Burkina Faso)

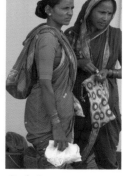
(India)

People in traditional cultures carry objects with their arms somewhat externally rotated (thumbs facing forward) or very externally rotated (palms facing forward.)

fig.6-16

fig.6-18

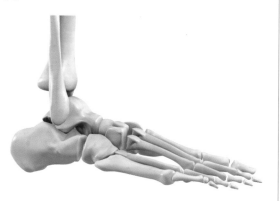

The heel bone in our species is a sturdy bone adapted for weight-bearing. The bones in the front of the foot, by contrast are delicate and not constructed to bear the weight of the body.

NATURAL ARCHES OF THE FEET

Tallstanding gives your arches (inner, outer, and transverse) a chance of staying intact (fig.6-19). Collapsed arches usually reflect significant postural distortion throughout the body, and they also cause a set of problems of their own, especially in the bones, joints, and ligaments of the feet. Flat feet appear to be far more common now than in earlier times, when they were considered enough of a disability to make a man unfit for military service. Now, flat feet are so common that the military cannot afford to exclude people on this basis.

WEIGHT ON THE HEELS

When we evolved from being quadrupedal to bipedal, the foot changed significantly. In comparing our feet with those of our primarily quadrupedal primate relatives, one of the striking differences is the sturdiness of the human heel bone. The bones towards the front of our feet remain relatively delicate, but the heel bone is enlarged and constructed with cross grain reinforcement for weight-bearing (fig.6-18). In our bones we have compelling evidence of how we are designed to stand: primarily on our heels.

fig.6-19

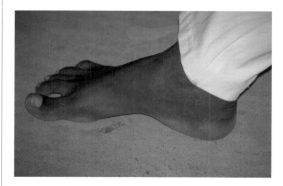

Healthy foot with intact arches (Brazil)

BARE FEET

A frequent question is whether it is healthy to go without shoes. The answer depends on the condition of your arch muscles, the alignment of your body, and the surface on which you stand and walk. If your feet and alignment are healthy, going barefoot on softer surfaces, such as grass, dirt, or sand, gives your foot muscles a healthy workout. If you have weak arch muscles, even a casual stroll on the beach can further distend your ligaments. Don't go barefoot without maintaining your weight over your heels and actively engaging your arch muscles while walking (see Lesson 8, Glidewalking). Even if your arches are in good shape, it is never advisable to go barefoot for any length of time on hard surfaces such as concrete or asphalt.

PREGNANCY

Pregnancy is a time when it is especially important to have healthy posture. Pregnant women are prone to damaging the ligaments in their feet. The hormone relaxin, circulating through their system to relax the pelvic joints in preparation for delivery, relaxes all ligaments, including those in the feet. The additional weight of the baby, especially if carried on the front of the feet, can permanently overstretch the foot ligaments. Some women experience a dramatic increase in foot length, sometimes as much as one or two sizes.

INSOLES

For people with flat arches, it is useful and, in fact, important to use an insole. The foot muscles cannot (and should not) always maintain the shape of the feet. When these muscles are relaxed, healthy ligaments fulfill this role. However, when foot ligaments are overstretched, an insole can provide the necessary support and prevent your foot from spreading. Select an insole that supports all three arches of the foot. Used passively, it will prevent further distortion of your foot. Used as a training device, it can remind you to use your foot muscles to maintain your arches.

Most commercial arch supports provide some protection and support for the most important arch of the foot, the inner arch. If you have little or no arch on the inner edge of your foot, commercially available arch supports may be adequate at first.

However, after a few months of doing the foot-strengthening exercises in Appendix 1, you should probably supplement these supports with an extra thickness of shaped rubber available at many shoe stores. The outer and transverse arches should also have support. To obtain arch supports that help with all three arches, you may have to look a little harder, or have them custom-made. Transverse arch supports, also called metatarsal arch supports, are often sold separately as pieces to be attached to a shoe, insole, or arch support.

Some podiatrists prescribe custom "orthotics." These tend to be fairly rigid and fairly expensive, and are usually constructed to reflect the existing shape of the patient's foot. This assumes that the shape of the foot will not change through time. In fact, there is a lot that people can and should do to modify their foot shape. For specifics, see the foot exercises in Appendix 1.

SHOES

Good shoes are especially important, given the harsh and unnatural surfaces on which we walk, and the corresponding damage and under-development in our feet. Unfortunately, good shoes are hard to find. Most consumers and many manufacturers are ignorant of what constitutes a good shoe, with the result that there is a proliferation of cheap and/or compromised footwear on the market. Here are some characteristics of a good shoe (fig.6-20):
- A firm last that provides a slight kidney-bean shape
- Shock-absorbent soles, particularly in the heel
- Arch supports for all three arches of the feet

SPINE CONTOUR CONFUSION

As a novice posture student, you may wonder why the profiles of certain muscular individuals (including a lot of Greek statues), that otherwise exhibit good posture, appear to be rounded in the upper spine (fig.6-21). These individuals have large muscles around their shoulders. Because the shoulders are placed back along the spine where they belong, they give the appearance of a rounded upper back. Yet the spine, buried especially deeply between the shoulder blades, remains straight.

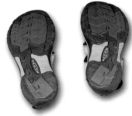
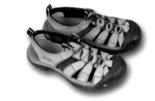
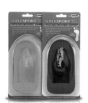

*Well-designed shoes have a kidney-bean shaped last,
pronounced arch supports, and shock-absorbent soles.*

*Well-designed insoles support the inner,
outer, and transverse arches of the foot.*

fig.6-21

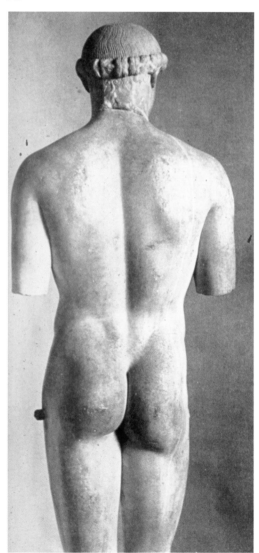
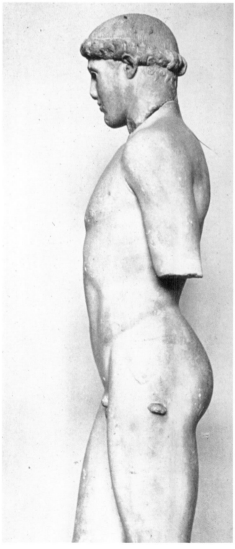

© Gerard Mackworth-Young

The straight thoracic spine is hidden behind large upper back muscles in these statues.

fig.6-22

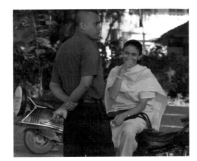

(India)

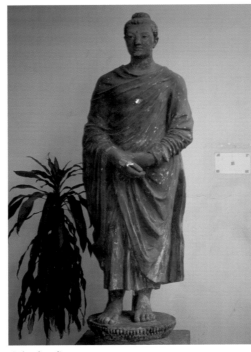

(Thailand)

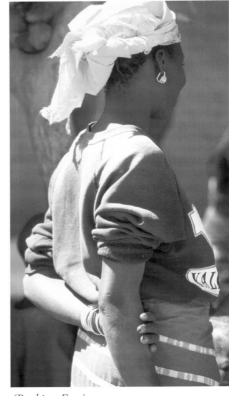

(Burkina Faso)

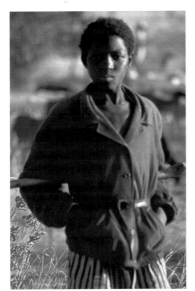

(Burkina Faso)

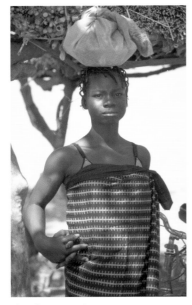

(Burkina Faso)

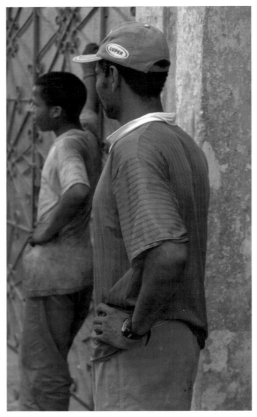

(Brazil)

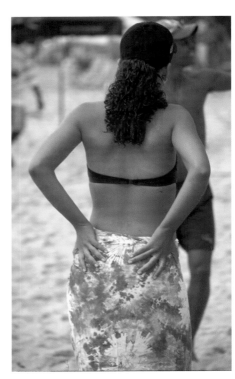

(Brazil)

People in traditional cultures often rest their arms on some part of their bodies.

RECAP

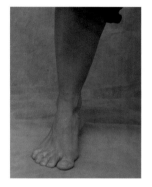

a. Form a kidney-bean shape with each foot

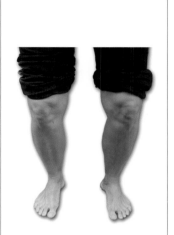

b. Rotate legs outward

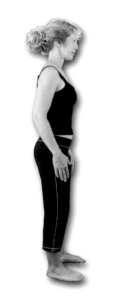

c. Shift most of your weight to your heels

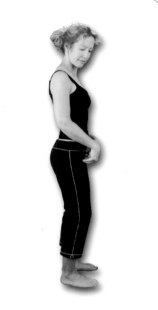

d. Soften knees and groin area, and tip pelvis forward

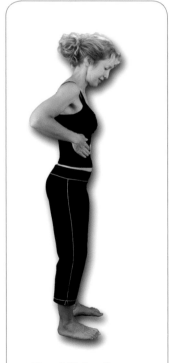

e. Establish rib anchor, if necessary

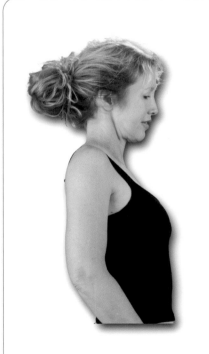

f. Perform shoulder roll with each shoulder

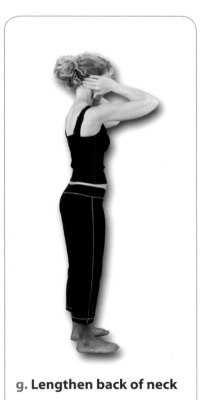

g. Lengthen back of neck

7

HIP-HINGING

Hinging at the hips to bend

This older Burkina woman was gathering water chestnuts while I photographed and filmed her for hours. She spends most of the time bent over, rising every 10 – 15 minutes for a very short time and then going back to her bent position. She does this every day for seven to nine hours and reports no pathology in her back (though she says she would prefer to sit in a chair all day!). Notice her flat back, the even groove overlying her spine, the well-developed musculature alongside her spine, and her shoulder blades positioned back and down relative to her spine (the same as they would be in standing).

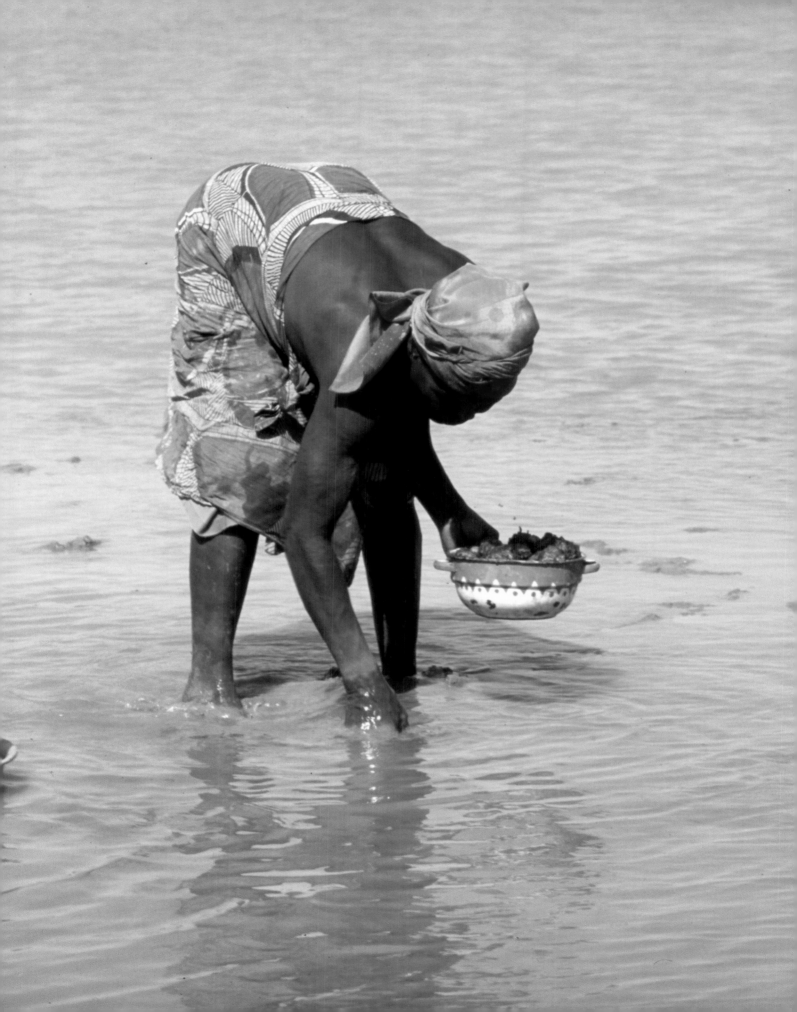

If there is one action that makes or breaks a back, it is bending. People who bend well usually enjoy good back health (fig.7-1); people who bend poorly often develop back pain (fig.7-2). Furthermore, by watching people bend, a skilled observer can predict where tension or pain is likely to occur (fig.7-3).

To learn how to bend well, we need to observe what people are doing in rural India or village Africa, as they bend over their rice paddies or gather water chestnuts all day (fig.7-5). These people can bend for long hours without a problem, while many of us in industrialized cultures cannot bend for even five minutes without pain.

fig.7-1

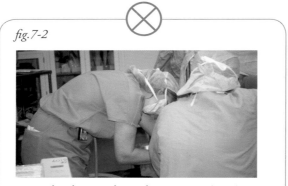

Woman bending well while washing clothes (Burkina Faso)

fig.7-4

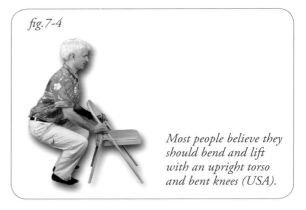

Most people believe they should bend and lift with an upright torso and bent knees (USA).

⊗

fig.7-2

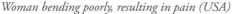

Woman bending poorly, resulting in pain (USA)

fig.7-5

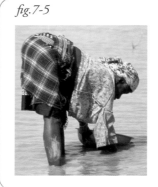

Example of healthy bending from the hips with straight knees and back (Burkina Faso).

⊗

fig.7-3

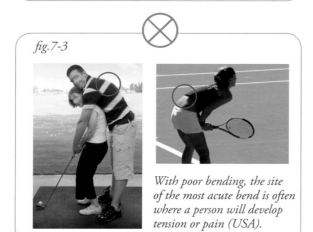

With poor bending, the site of the most acute bend is often where a person will develop tension or pain (USA).

Of all our common daily activities, bending is the one that is least often done right, and the one that most experts teach inadequately (fig.7-4).

Successful bending requires a healthy baseline back contour that you preserve as you bend. By now, you have achieved that baseline:

• You have learned to tip your pelvis forward in anteversion to restore your natural lumbo-sacral angle.
• You have lengthened the muscles that run longitudinally on either side of your spine so they no longer draw your spine into the shape of an over-strung bow.
• You have reset your shoulder blades further back so their weight and the weight of your arms no longer curve your spine forward.
• You have resettled your head further back to crown the spine so that its weight no longer causes your upper spine to curve forward.
• You have learned to use your abdominal muscles of your inner corset to preserve

the natural shape of your spine and, when necessary, lengthen it.

In this lesson, you will learn how to bend without undoing all that fine work.

ANATOMY OF A BACKACHE...

Most people round their backs as they bend, compressing the front (anterior) part of certain discs and squeezing the contents to the back (posterior) part (fig.7-6). This causes wear on the fibrous exterior at the back of the disc, the worst possible site. Because the spinal cord and emerging nerves lie directly behind the discs, a disc that bulges or herniates in the posterior direction is likely to impinge on the nerves behind it, causing pain, numbness, tingling, and loss of muscle function anywhere along the pathway of that nerve.

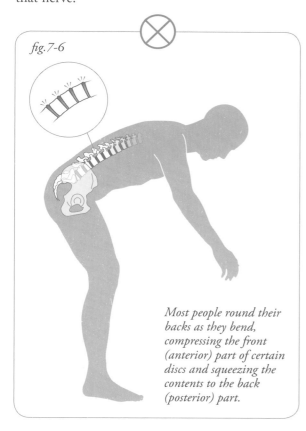

fig.7-6

Most people round their backs as they bend, compressing the front (anterior) part of certain discs and squeezing the contents to the back (posterior) part.

In addition, rounding the back stretches some of the ligaments in the rounded part. Since ligaments are not elastic, repeated stretching at the same site can cause them to become lax and lose their function of limiting spinal distortion. Ligament distension can result in abnormal forward

curvature (*kyphosis*) even when standing upright (fig.7-7). An extreme case is the "dowager's hump," where flaccid ligaments permit an extreme curvature in the thoracic spine.

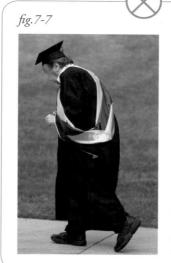

fig.7-7

Overstretched ligaments around the spine can lead to abnormal spinal curvature (USA).

... AND HOW TO AVOID IT

Healthy bending involves hinging at the hip joint rather than elsewhere in the torso, preserving the shape and length of the back throughout the bend. The advantages of bending this way are many. No discs are compromised and no back ligaments are strained. The knees are spared and the back muscles benefit from a healthy challenge. Whereas improper bending is indeed a threat to the back, healthy bending through hip-hinging is a beneficial exercise.

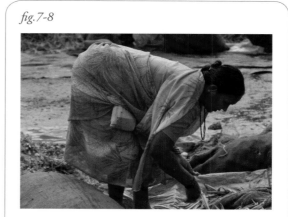

fig.7-8

Hip-hinging provides healthy exercise for muscles and spares joints (India).

With hip-hinging, the *erector spinae* muscles work to keep the back aligned, rather than rounded forward in response to the pull of gravity (fig.7-9). This strengthens the muscles and is, in fact, an ideal way to train them: the different fibers of the muscles develop exactly as needed to keep the back straight.

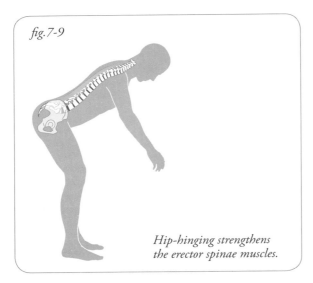

fig.7-9

Hip-hinging strengthens the erector spinae muscles.

Hip-hinging stretches the hamstring muscles with every bend (fig.7-10). Indeed, periodic bending increases flexibility in these muscles, which is key to healthy pelvic anteversion. In contrast, tight hamstrings pull on the sitz bones (*ischial tuberosities*), forcing the pelvis into retroversion (fig.7-11). Note that if your hamstrings are tight, you can ease the demands on them by bending your knees as needed. But don't bend your knees unnecessarily, as this puts undue pressure on the knee joints.

fig.7-11

⊗

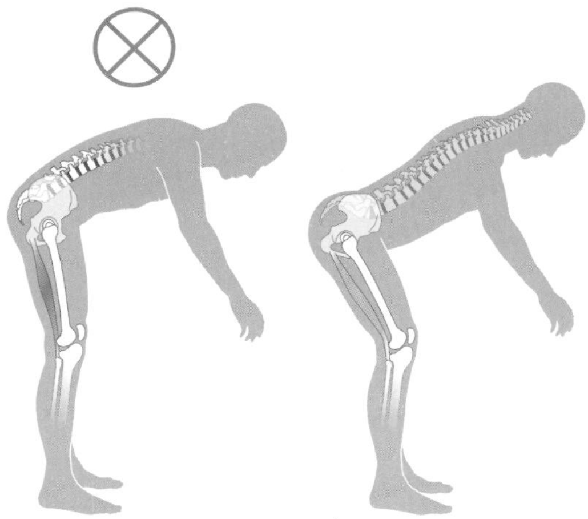

a.   b.

a) Tight hamstring muscles pull on the sitz bones (ischial tuberosities), making it difficult to tip the pelvis forward for hip-hinging. b) Bending the knees compensates for tight hamstring muscles and facilitates hip-hinging.

When you bend well, the rhomboid muscles, which run between the inner borders of the shoulder blades and the thoracic spine, work to prevent the shoulder blades from slumping forward (fig.7-12). The extra strength they develop during bending helps their resting function. The stronger and more toned they are, the better they can peg your shoulder blades back and in toward your spine. In a modern lifestyle, there are not many opportunities to strengthen the rhomboids, as we do not draw water from wells or haul in fishnets. Bending well is one of the few ways of challenging these muscles.

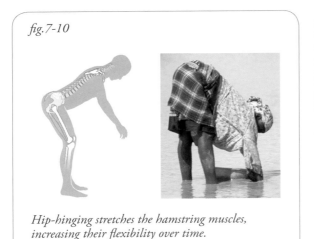

fig.7-10

Hip-hinging stretches the hamstring muscles, increasing their flexibility over time.

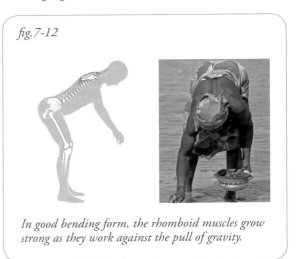

fig.7-12

In good bending form, the rhomboid muscles grow strong as they work against the pull of gravity.

People are often taught to bend with their knees to preserve their backs. Although this does preserve the back, it stresses the knees a great deal, and eliminates opportunities to lengthen the hamstring muscles and strengthen the back muscles (fig.7-13). It is also impractical for many tasks. You should reserve bending with your knees for those tasks that would over-challenge your back muscles (for example, when lifting objects that are unusually heavy) and for when your back is injured.

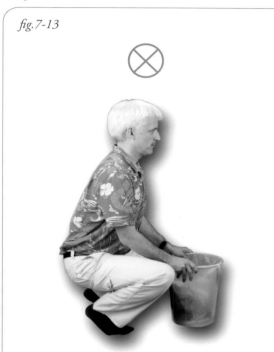

fig.7-13

a. *The way to bend that is usually recommended can cause excessive wear and tear to the knees and is impractical for many tasks (USA).*

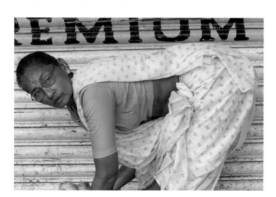

b. *Hip-hinging spares the knees and is very practical (India).*

BENEFITS

- Avoids compressing or compromising the spinal discs

- Avoids distending the ligaments around the spine

- Strengthens key back muscles

- Stretches hamstring muscles

- Strengthens rhomboid muscles

COMPARING DIFFERENT BENDING STYLES

The following table summarizes the positive and negative effects of three bending styles. Hip-hinging is the only style that has no negative effects.

EFFECT ON	HIP-HINGING	BENDING WITH A ROUNDED BACK	BENDING WITH THE KNEES
DISCS	Preserves	Damages	Preserves
LIGAMENTS	Preserves	Distends	Preserves
KNEES	Preserves	Preserves	Wears
BACK MUSCLES	Strengthens	Does not strengthen; perhaps stretches	No effect
HAMSTRINGS	Stretches	Minimal to no stretch	No effect
RHOMBOIDS	Strengthens	Does not strengthen; perhaps stretches	No effect

With young children at home, I got fed up with picking things up around the house. I didn't want to bend any more. It was uncomfortable. Hip-hinging was a revelation. This kind of bending was comfortable and had the extra benefit of stretching the hamstrings. It actually felt energizing. Now I also hip-hinge when I garden, and it gives my knees a break.

Madeleine de Corwin, retired Canadian M.D., Palo Alto, CA

EQUIPMENT

You will need a full-length mirror.

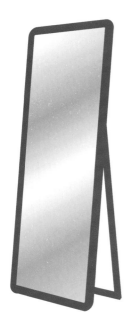

PREPARING FOR A DEEP BEND

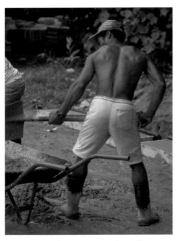

Notice wide stance and well-aligned legs (Brazil)

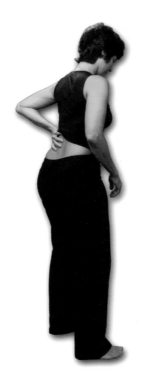

1 STAND WITH YOUR FEET POINTED OUTWARD ABOUT 10°-15° WITH EACH IN A KIDNEY-BEAN SHAPE

To bend just a little, place your feet about hip-width apart. To bend deeply, use a wider stance.

2 PLACE ONE HAND ON YOUR LOW BACK WITH THE FINGERTIPS ON YOUR MIDLINE GROOVE

This hand will monitor your groove as you bend.

3 SOFTEN YOUR KNEES; DO NOT LOCK THEM

This allows your knees to bend as needed to accommodate tight hamstrings.

4 START TO BEND YOUR TORSO FORWARD FROM THE HIP JOINTS

Feel your pelvis rotate forward on the heads of the thigh bones (*femurs*). Your pelvis leads and your back follows. When the pelvis stops moving, the back stops moving. Your fingertips should feel no change to your midline groove. If you feel the groove disappear or deepen, straighten up and proceed again with care. See pages 162-163 for more detailed guidance.

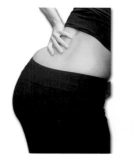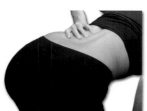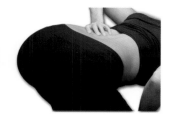

Hip-hinging with a healthy back

IDEAL AND COMPROMISED WAYS TO BEND

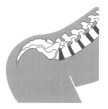

Hip-hinging exercises the back muscles and does not threaten the discs.

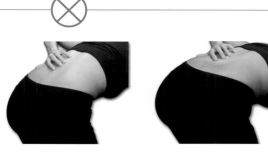

Bending with a rounded back

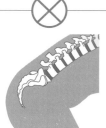

Rounding the back while bending compresses the spinal discs in a particularly dangerous way.

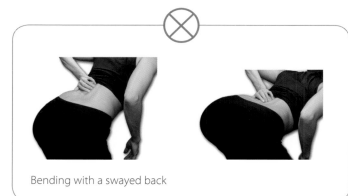

Bending with a swayed back

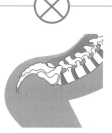

Swaying while bending generally compresses the spine.

DEGREE OF HAMSTRING FLEXIBILITY INFLUENCES BENDING FORM

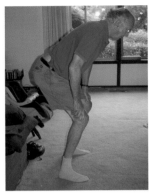

Limited hamstring flexibility necessitates significant bending with the knees while hip-hinging (USA).

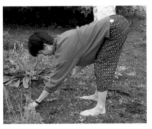

Good hamstring flexibility permits hip-hinging with slight bending at the knees (USA).

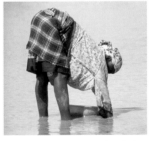

Extreme hamstring flexibility allows for hip-hinging with straight legs (Burkina Faso).

5 IF YOUR HAMSTRINGS ARE TIGHT, BEND YOUR KNEES AS NEEDED TO PRESERVE THE SHAPE OF YOUR BACK

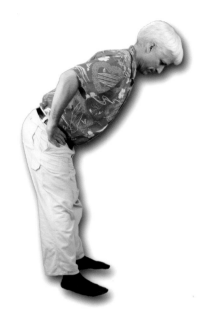

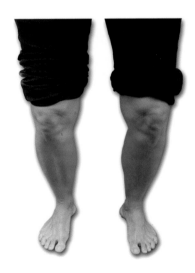

Be sure the knees point in the same direction as the feet, and the bend is smooth and coordinated.

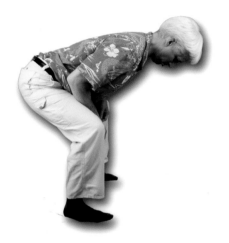

A common mistake is to let the knees turn in. Fashioning the feet into a more exaggerated kidney-bean shape usually solves this problem. Some people may find it necessary to also use their leg muscles to rotate their legs outward and align their knees.

6 DURING THE BEND, KEEP YOUR HEAD, NECK, AND SHOULDERS IN THE SAME RELATIONSHIP TO YOUR TORSO AS WHEN STANDING UPRIGHT

Think of your neck as an extension of your spine. Engage the muscles at the back of the neck to keep your head and neck from protruding forward. Engage the rhomboid muscles to prevent your shoulders from slumping forward.

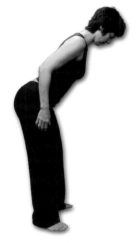

a.

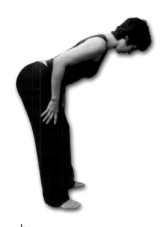

b.

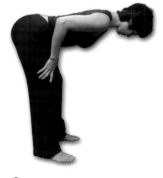

c.

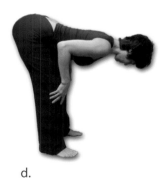

d.

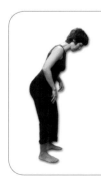

A common mistake is to let your head and/or shoulders protrude forward, breaking the upper body alignment.

ARABESK BIRD

This familiar toy provides a useful image to help you hip-hinge.

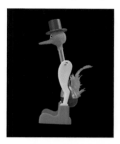

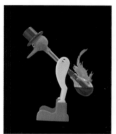

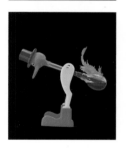

MECHANICAL TOYS

Old-fashioned mechanical toys often exhibit a traditional bending form.

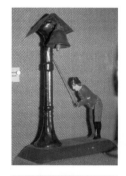

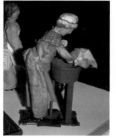

"BIRD'S BEAK"

Nesting the pelvis between the legs results in an acute angle between the legs and torso, called a "bird's beak" in Portuguese culture.

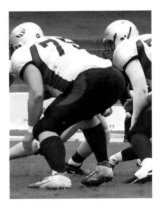

Football player in line of scrimmage (USA)

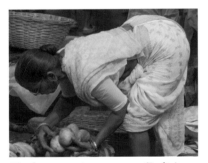

Vendor arranging mangoes (India)

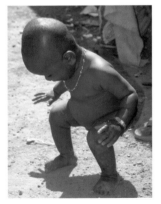

This childs' pelvis and belly nest easily between his legs (Burkina Faso).

7 AS YOU GO INTO A DEEPER BEND, NEST THE PELVIS BETWEEN THE LEGS

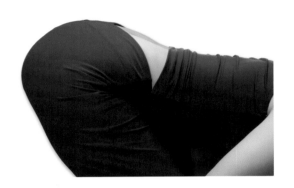

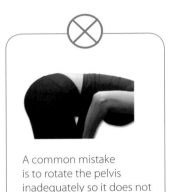

A common mistake is to rotate the pelvis inadequately so it does not nest between the legs

This can only happen if the legs are externally rotated and there is some flexibility in the hip joint. If you cannot find this action now, skip it. As you increase flexibility around your hip joints, the action becomes easier (see Appendix 1 for an optional stretch to accelerate this process).

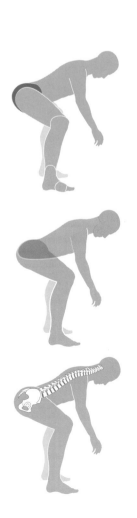

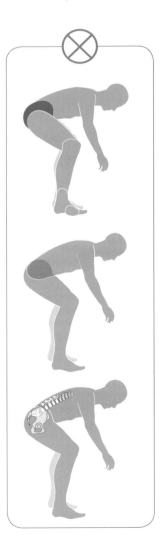

8 WHEN YOU ARE READY TO STRAIGHTEN UP, UNHINGE AT THE HIP JOINT, MOVING THE TORSO AS ONE UNIT

Monitor your groove with your fingertips as you do this. Once again, your goal is to maintain the same groove depth throughout the action.

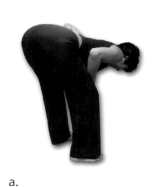

a.

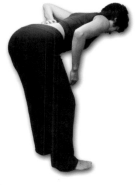

b.

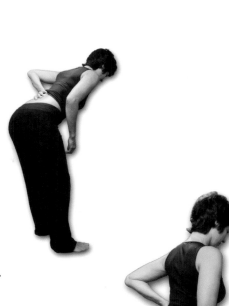

c.

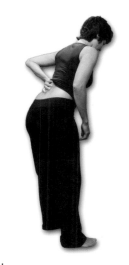

d.

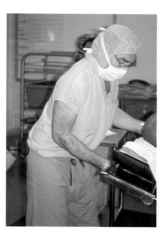

e.

EXAMPLES OF STRAIGHT BACKS WITH HIP-HINGING

As these people bend and unbend, their backs remain straight.

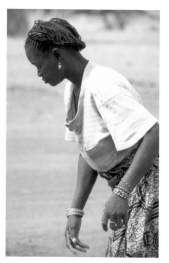

Young woman (Burkina Faso)

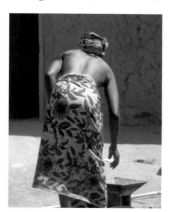

Older woman (Burkina Faso)

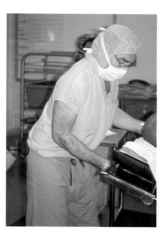

Surgeon (USA)

INDICATIONS OF IMPROVEMENT

At first hip-hinging may require concentration and slow motion. With time you will memorize this movement pattern and be able to do it as quickly and automatically as your old way of bending.

The muscle strength and flexibility you create by hip-hinging will in turn facilitate improved bending form. Over time you will find it easier to bend deeply, stay in a bent position longer, and bend your knees less (fig.7-14). As you perfect the form and combine it with engaging your inner corset (see Lesson 5), you will feel confident about combining bending and lifting (fig.7-15).

fig.7-14

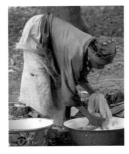

Hip-hinging will allow you to bend deeper, for longer periods of time, with straighter legs (Burkina Faso).

fig.7-15

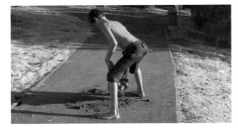

With practice, you will gain the confidence to lift heavier objects while hip-hinging. Do not attempt this before your form is excellent.

TROUBLESHOOTING

BENDING IS PAINFUL

Perhaps your back muscles are in spasm from a recent injury. Because this way of bending uses your back muscles, it may be better to bend using just your knees until your back is further healed. Perhaps the pain is caused by rounding or swaying your back as you bend. If so, try engaging your inner corset before you begin to bend. This helps you maintain your torso as a single unit. If you are still having trouble, bend with your knees until you perfect your technique.

THE GROOVE IN YOUR LOW BACK DISAPPEARS AS YOU BEND

This problem is very common when people are learning to hip-hinge. It is difficult (for some people, very difficult) to rotate the pelvis forward as a part of bending. It takes patience. Keep in mind that you have a deeply ingrained subroutine in your brain that is triggered when you bend. You are now trying to edit this subroutine.

Place your fingertips on your midline groove to give you feedback as you very slowly try to bend by rotating your pelvis forward. If you feel any change in the groove, return to the point where the groove is restored. Practice bending just a little way while keeping your groove intact. Soon you will be able to bend further with your groove intact. Looking at your profile in a mirror is another way to get useful feedback. It sometimes helps to reach back and around to your sitz bones and pull them up to help this action (fig.7-16).

Remember that tight hamstrings might limit how far forward you can bend with straight legs without loosing your groove. An easy solution is to bend the knees as needed. Tight *external hip rotator* muscles can restrict your pelvis from nesting between the legs, causing the back to round during a deep bend. In both cases, exercises to lengthen the muscles are beneficial. See Appendix 1 for exercises that target these muscles.

fig.7-16

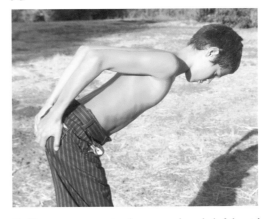

Pulling up on your sitz bones can be a helpful guide to tipping your pelvis forward into anteversion.

THE GROOVE IN YOUR LOW BACK GETS DEEPER AS YOU BEND

As you bend, the demands on your back muscles increase to resist the pull of gravity. Ideally, the *erector spinae* muscles contract just enough to keep the shape of your spine constant throughout your bend. If the muscles overcompensate, the groove in your back deepens. You may be contracting the muscles of your low back out of habit. It takes patience and feedback from your fingertips to eliminate this tension from your bending routine.

If you still cannot keep the groove from deepening, try to engage your inner corset as you bend (see Lesson 5). This will help you move your torso as a unit and learn the new movement pattern. Later, when you have learned the pattern, you will no longer need to use your inner corset for normal bending, but can reserve it for when you need to lift heavy objects.

FURTHER INFORMATION

In this lesson you have learned the ideal way to bend with no distortion in the back. A healthy back can accommodate small distortions in bending, particularly in the upper *(thoracic)* spine, without incurring damage. The shape of the lumbar spine, however, should not change throughout the bend.

HAMSTRING FLEXIBILITY

Village African women, who spend long hours bending or sitting with outstretched legs (fig. 7-17), tend to have especially flexible hamstring muscles and frequently bend with completely flat backs (figs.7-1, 7-5). The men, who spend less time in these two positions, have less hamstring flexibility and often round their thoracic spines slightly as they bend. They do, however, preserve a healthy shape in their lumbar spines (fig.7-18).

The degree of flexibility in the hamstring muscles also dictates how much the knees must bend to preserve a straight back in hip-hinging (see photos on page 158).

fig.7-17

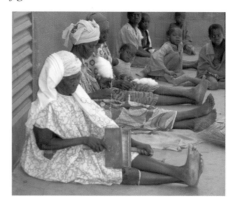

Weavers spend many hours sitting with outstretched legs, resulting in very flexible hamstring muscles (Burkina Faso).

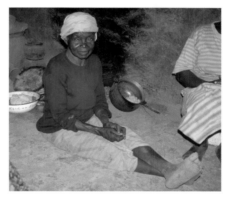

Flexible hamstring muscles are one result of doing household chores while sitting with outstretched legs (Burkina Faso).

fig.7-18

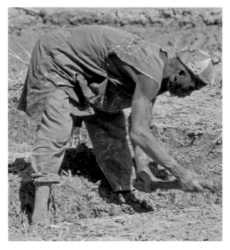

A slightly less "perfect" bending form that includes some curvature in the thoracic, but not the lumbar, spine (Burkina Faso).

BENDING FOR EXTENDED PERIODS

When bending for long periods of time, as when weeding a garden, it is natural to rest a forearm, elbow or hand on the corresponding thigh (fig.7-20). This is more restful for your back muscles.

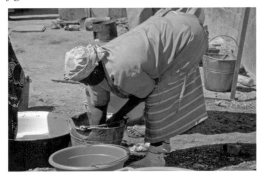

fig.7-20

Resting a forearm on a thigh facilitates hip-hinging for an extended period (Burkina Faso).

BENDING WHILE SITTING

The same principles for bending apply whether sitting or standing (fig.7-21).

fig.7-21

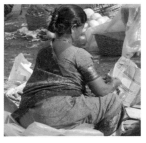

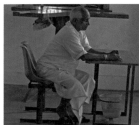

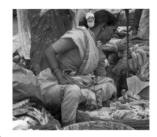

These people hip-hinge well while sitting (India).

EXTRA WEIGHT

Full-bodied people often bend well (fig.7-22), perhaps because the downside of bending poorly would be extreme and immediate.

fig.7-22

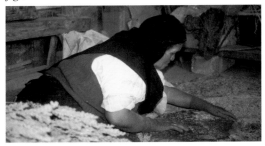

This full-bodied woman has excellent bending technique (Ecuador).

HIP-HINGING FOR ATHLETIC ADVANTAGE

Hip-hinging puts your entire body in a position of mechanical advantage to optimize performance in most sports. The shoulders remain in their baseline position, increasing the range of motion of the arms and optimizing the blood circulation to and from the arms. The pelvis is anteverted, putting the muscles in the lower limbs in a position of mechanical advantage. In addition, hip-hinging is easy on your joints, enabling you to play your sport with fewer injuries for more years.

The photo below (fig. 7-23) shows my son on the right winning a Bay Area wrestling tournament over from an opponent widely regarded as stronger than he. Notice that his form gives him more reach, better arm position and better buttock position, all of which are important in most sports.

fig.7-23

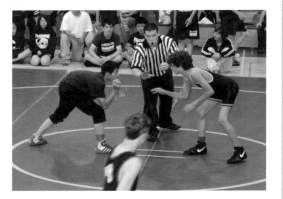

Hip-hinging offers advantages in athletic performance.

TRAINING CHILDREN TO HIP-HINGE

It is important to handle infants in ways that preserve the alignment of their spines (see figs. F-13 and F-14 on pages 13-14). Doing so helps the child learn to use the torso as a unit (fig. 7-24), rather than distort it too readily when performing actions with the arms or legs. Additionally, providing good models helps children develop and maintain healthy movement patterns.

fig.7-24

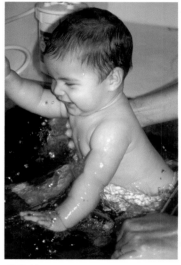

(USA)

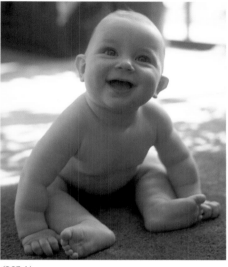

(USA)

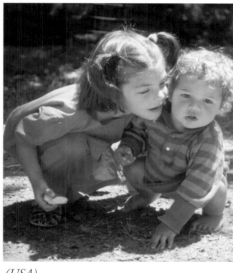

(USA)

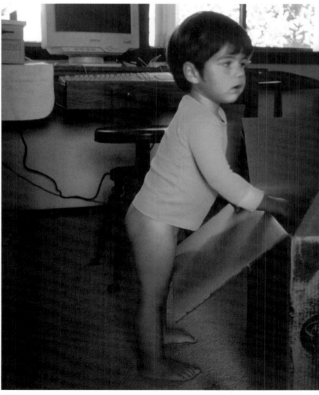

(USA)

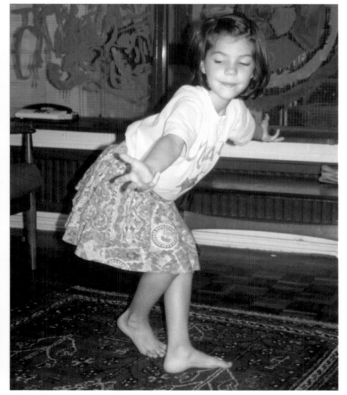

(USA)

Babies that have been carried and handled well tend to bend by hip-hinging.

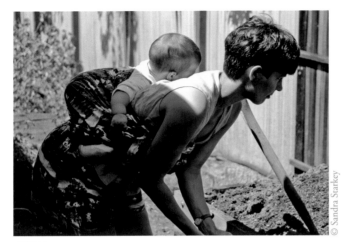

(USA)

© Sandra Starkey

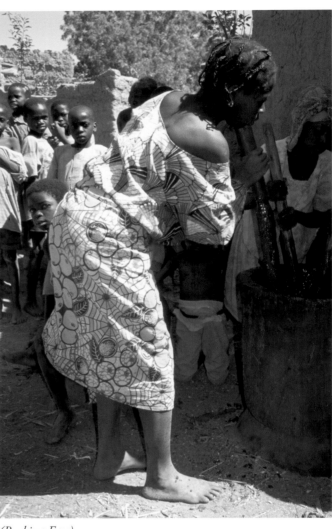

(Burkina Faso)

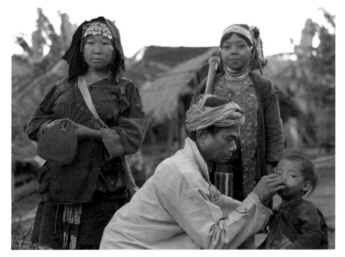

(Thailand)

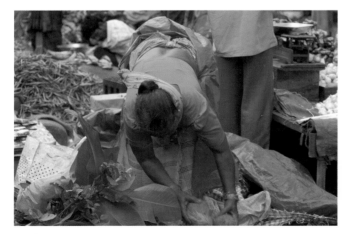

(India)

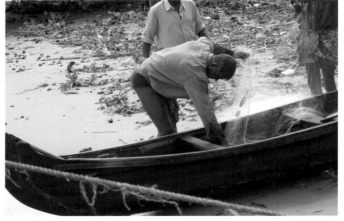

(India)

RECAP

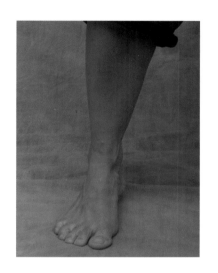

a. Form a kidney-bean shape with each foot

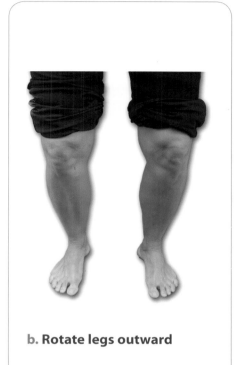

b. Rotate legs outward

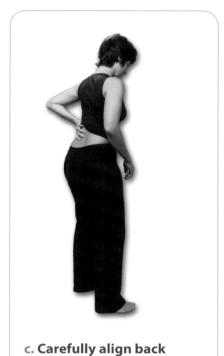

c. Carefully align back

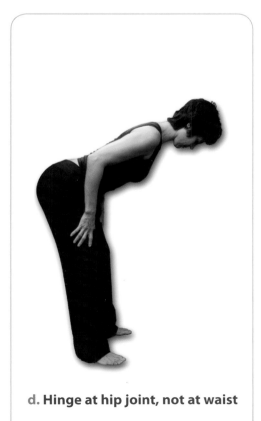

d. Hinge at hip joint, not at waist

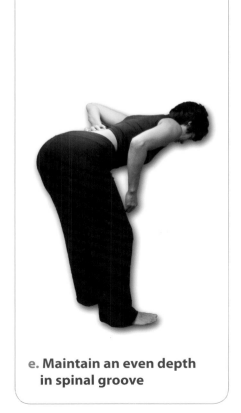

e. Maintain an even depth in spinal groove

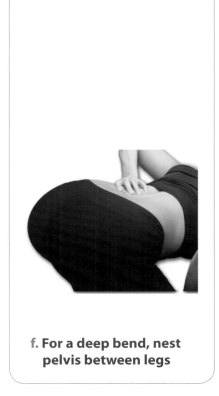

f. For a deep bend, nest pelvis between legs

8

GLIDEWALKING

Walking as a series of forward propulsions, not falls

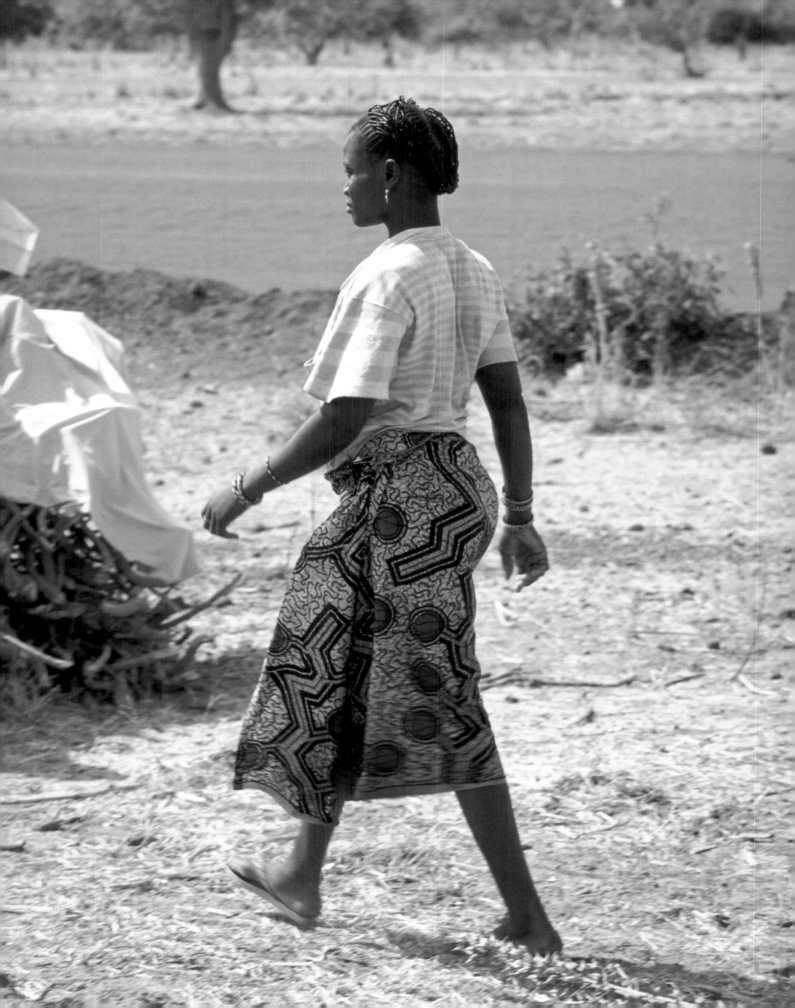

In this lesson, you will learn to walk well. Walking is often hailed as one of the best exercises you can do, and it is! A brisk walk, when done in a healthful way, provides excellent cardio-vascular exercise. It also tones and stretches muscles in your lower body with a relatively low risk of injury to joints, bones, or muscles (fig.8-1).

If you walk poorly, however, you may under-use some muscles and over-use your joints, risking injury and degeneration. For many people in industrial cultures, walking consists of a series of forward falls blocked abruptly by the forward leg. The gluteal and leg muscles are under-used (fig.8-2, 8-3). The back twists, sways, or hunches as it jerks with each step. The impact of each step is an assault to every weight-bearing joint in the body.

fig.8-2

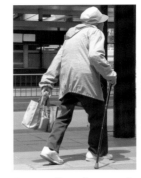

Poor walking form predisposes the hip joint to wear and tear, and under-exercises the leg and buttock muscles.

fig.8-3

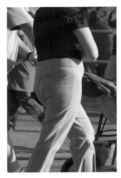

(USA) *(France)*

Poor walking form is so prevalent in industrial societies that even our traffic signs show bad form.

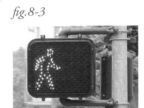
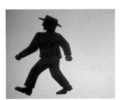

(Bulgaria) *(Italy)*

In countries with intact kinesthetic traditions, traffic signs correspondingly exhibit good walking form.

fig.8-1

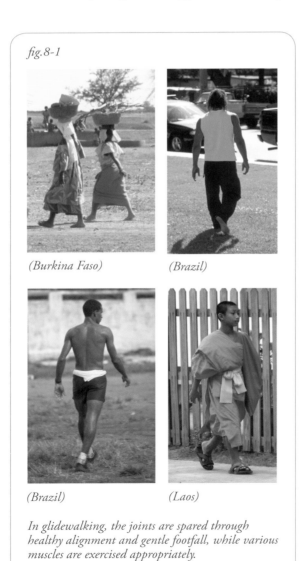

(Burkina Faso) *(Brazil)*

(Brazil) *(Laos)*

In glidewalking, the joints are spared through healthy alignment and gentle footfall, while various muscles are exercised appropriately.

Walking should be a series of controlled forward propulsions. The buttock and leg muscles contract strongly to propel the body forward, thus getting the exercise they need while the back is spared unnecessary wear and tear. The torso is stable and moves forward smoothly while the buttocks, legs, and feet do the work. The arms and shoulders are relatively still unless you are walking very briskly. The overall sensation is that of gliding forward through space. This way of walking has become rare enough in our society to deserve a special name: glidewalking.

One of the benefits of glidewalking is that it strengthens the buttock (*gluteus*) muscles (fig.8-4). Strong gluteus muscles support pelvic anteversion, which is key to healthy posture. Strong gluteus muscles also play an important role in keeping one's balance and preventing falls. In most people in industrialized cultures, the gluteus muscles are underdeveloped. This is especially problematic in elderly people, who have a high risk of bone fracture when they fall.

fig.8-4

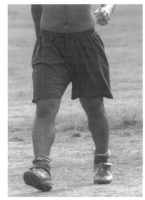

(Brazil)

Glidewalking strengthens the gluteus muscles; strong gluteus muscles support pelvic anteversion.

Glidewalking provides one of the few opportunities in daily activity to stretch the *psoas* muscle, which runs from the front of the lumbar spine to the upper inside of the thigh bone (*femur*). A tight psoas sways the low back and contributes to back pain. In glidewalking, the psoas gets a beneficial stretch at the moment of push-off (fig.8-5).

fig.8-5

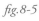

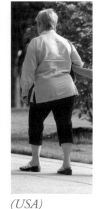

(India)   (USA)

Glidewalking stretches the psoas muscles.

Glidewalking also provides a good opportunity to strengthen the arch muscles of the feet. Most people walk in a way that only uses the large muscles of the leg. Ideally, walking also uses the foot arch muscles. If we walked barefoot on natural surfaces, the arch muscles would strengthen as the feet worked to grab and push off the ground. Because of the prevalence of shoes and man-made surfaces, most people use the muscles of their feet merely as padding. In glidewalking, the arch muscles are actively engaged with each step (fig.8-6). This is parallel to skilled cycling where, in addition to the large leg muscles, the arch muscles of the feet augment the power of each "stride."

fig.8-6

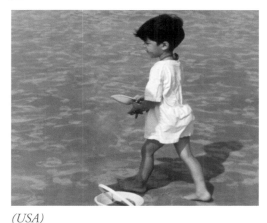

(USA)

Glidewalking strengthens the arch muscles of the foot; strong arch muscles maintain the baseline shape of the foot as a platform for the work of other muscles.

Glidewalking helps preserve the health of the hip joints in several ways. First, glidewalking strengthens the buttocks and stretches the psoas muscles, helping restore pelvic anteversion and normal architecture in the hip joints. Poor alignment in the hip joints and the resulting stiffness in the surrounding muscles predispose one to arthritis of the hip joints (fig.8-7). Restoring normal architecture in the hip joints stops this process from progressing further and can reverse some of the damage that has happened. Second, glidewalking includes a relaxed "swing phase" in each stride (fig.8-8), which helps restore a healthy joint space between the head of the thigh bone (*femur*) and the hip socket (*acetabulum*). Many people keep the muscles surrounding the hip joints tense at all times, causing stress within the hip joints.

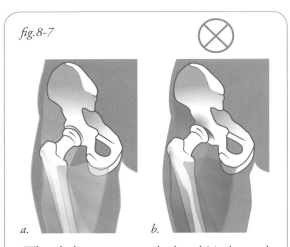

fig.8-7

a.   *b.*

When the hip joint is correctly aligned (a), the muscles around the joint can relax appropriately, there is adequate space within the joint, and the fit between the leg and hip bones is correct. With poor alignment at the hip joint (b), some of the surrounding muscles are obliged to remain tense, the space in the joint is jammed, and the poor fit between the leg and hip bones predisposes the joint to arthritic changes.

During the swing phase of glidewalking, the leg hangs like a pendulum from the hip socket, stretching these muscles. Third, the soft impact of glidewalking causes no damage to the hip or other weight-bearing joints. A heavy tread jams the hip joint (and every other weight-bearing joint) with every step. Glidewalking limits the amount of stress in the weight-bearing joints to a healthy level, sufficient to prevent osteoporosis but not so much as to cause wear or arthritic changes.

fig.8-8

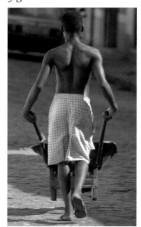 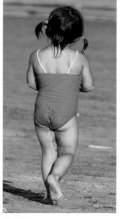

(Brazil)   *(USA)*

With glidewalking, the leg hangs loosely from the hip socket in the swing phase, re-establishing a healthy space in the hip joint.

You will learn this new way of walking in increasing rounds of detail. You may feel you should be able to master all this in a single session, but most people cannot. Remember, it took you about a year to master walking when you first learned, and you started with a clean slate. Now you have to unlearn your old pattern before you can master this new way of locomotion. But it won't take forever, because this time you have your intellect to help, and you have explicit instructions.

BENEFITS

• Strengthens the gluteus muscles, improving balance and helping maintain pelvic anteversion

• Strengthens the leg muscles

• Stretches the psoas muscles

• Strengthens the arch muscles of the feet

• Restores and maintains healthy hip joints

• Provides appropriate stress to weight-bearing bones, helping to prevent osteoporosis

• Reduces excessive stress to weight-bearing joints, preventing wear and tear.

• Stimulates circulation throughout the body, especially in the legs, helping to prevent blood clots, varicose veins, and other problems

Studying this method has enabled me to avoid what would have been my fifth foot surgery. I can now walk again without pain. It has given me a new lease on life.

Honor Rautmann, business owner, Sun River, OR

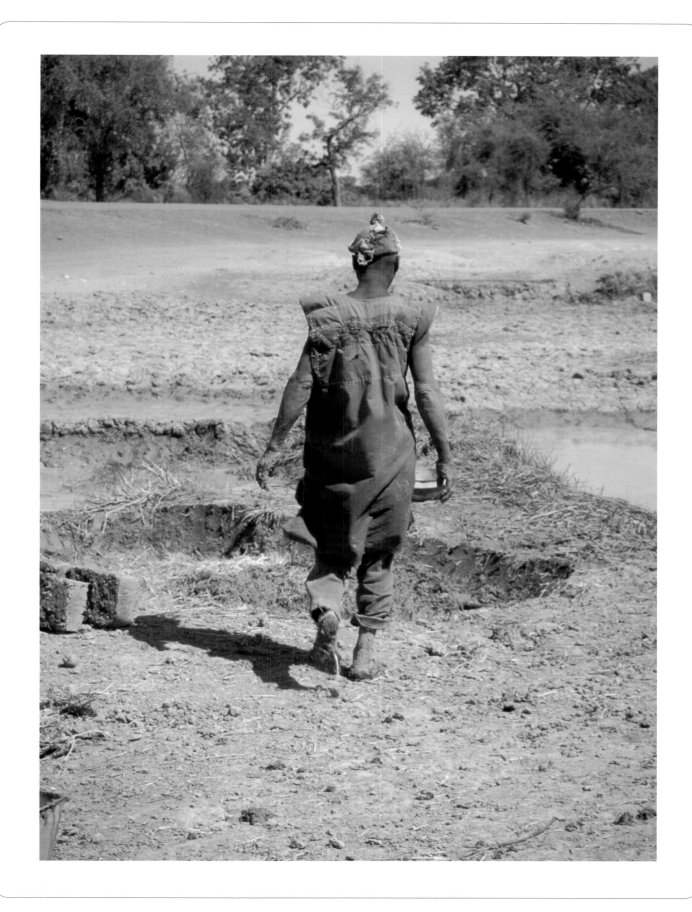

EQUIPMENT

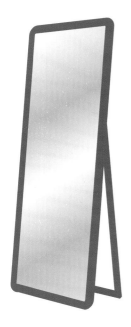

• *A full-length mirror*
• *A wall, table, or counter for balance*

PREPARING TO WALK

In this section you will learn movements that prepare you for the initiation, push-off, and swing phases of walking.

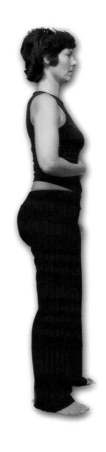

1 STAND WELL WITH AN ANTEVERTED PELVIS AND SOFT KNEES

Pelvic anteversion places your buttocks in a position of mechanical advantage, for a strong push-off in walking. Check that the back of your neck is elongated, your shoulders are rolled back, and the front lower edge of your rib cage is flush with your abdomen. For better balance, place one hand on a wall, table, or counter.

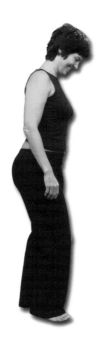

2 SHIFT YOUR WEIGHT ONTO YOUR LEFT LEG

Try to minimize disturbance to the rest of your body. In particular, keep the pelvis in a horizontal line from left to right.

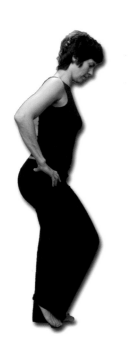

3 BEND YOUR RIGHT KNEE AND HINGE AT THE GROIN

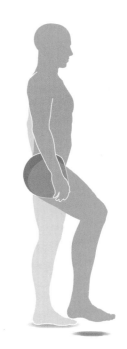

Don't tuck your pelvis or engage your quads. Allow your pelvis to settle further into anteversion to disengage your quads. This obliges your psoas muscle to perform the next action.

4 MOVE YOUR RIGHT LEG FORWARD AS THOUGH TO TAKE A STEP, BUT DO NOT PLACE YOUR FOOT ON THE FLOOR

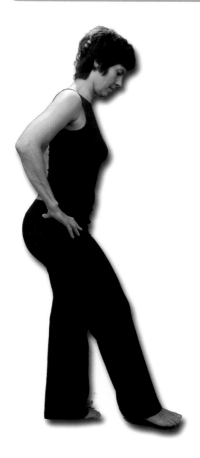

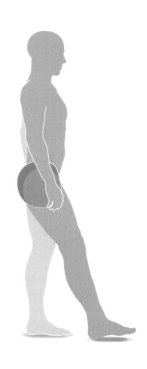

Again, do not tuck the pelvis or move the torso forward. If possible, stand in profile to a full-length mirror and monitor that your hips remain in place.

5 MOVE YOUR RIGHT LEG BACK, BENDING YOUR KNEE SO YOUR FOOT CLEARS THE FLOOR

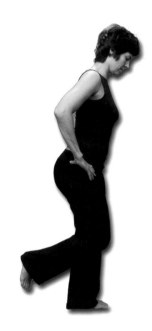

Make sure your foot clears the floor.

6 EXTEND YOUR RIGHT LEG BEHIND YOU, PLACING THE BALL OF THE FOOT ON THE FLOOR

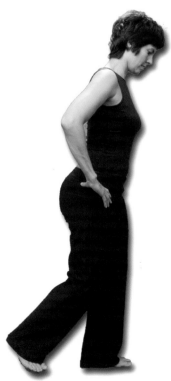

Do not extend your leg so far back that you shift your pelvis or torso. All the motion is in your hip joint. The toe of your right foot contacts the floor a little behind the left heel.

7 TIGHTEN YOUR RIGHT BUTTOCK, STRAIGHTEN YOUR RIGHT LEG, AND PRESS YOUR RIGHT HEEL TOWARDS THE FLOOR

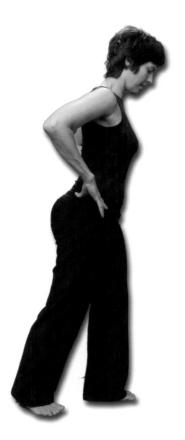

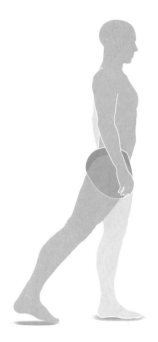

You should feel the gluteus medius muscle in your right buttock contract. If you have trouble locating this muscle, the exercise on page 213 will help you.

Tightening the buttock, straightening the leg, and pressing the heel towards the floor prepare you for glidewalking.

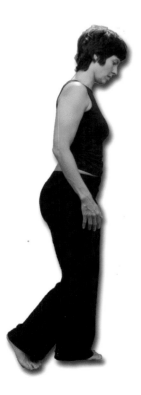

8 RELAX ALL THE MUSCLES IN THE RIGHT HIP AREA AND EASE THE LEG FORWARD, BUT LEAVE THE TIP OF THE BIG TOE ON THE GROUND

As the right leg drifts forward, allow it to hang freely from its socket. The right knee will come to rest beside the left knee.

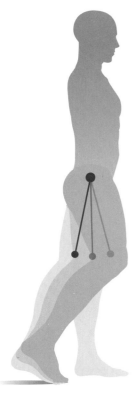

Relax the muscles around the hip joint so that the leg can dangle like a pendulum.

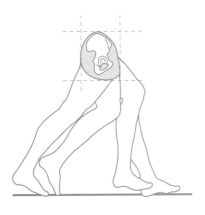

Note that the pelvis remains stationary as the leg moves forward and back

9 PLACE YOUR RIGHT HAND ON YOUR RIGHT THIGH AND GIVE A GENTLE PUSH

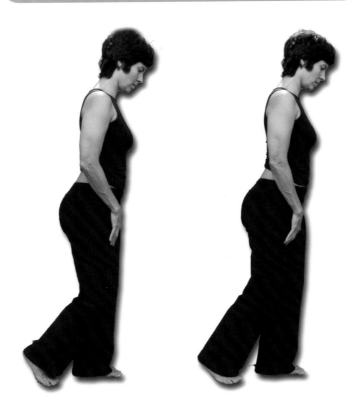

Your right leg should swing freely like a pendulum. If it does not, you have not succeeded in completely relaxing all the muscles.

10 REPEAT STEPS 3 THROUGH 9 SEVERAL TIMES WITH YOUR RIGHT LEG

Strive for a smooth leg motion without moving your torso.

11 STAND ON YOUR RIGHT LEG AND REPEAT THESE MOVEMENTS WITH YOUR LEFT LEG

Practice this sequence of movements until you can do it easily. You will incorporate it into your new way of walking. The forward movement resembles the initiation of every stride, the back movement resembles the push-off, and the pendulum movement resembles the swing phase.

GLIDEWALKING: FOCUSING ON THE WEIGHT-BEARING LEG

As you walk, each leg alternates between an active, weight-bearing phase and a passive, swing phase. When you practice the movements in this section, focus your attention on the weight-bearing leg.

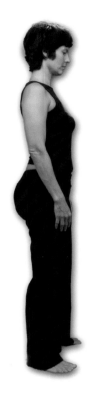

1 AS IN THE PREVIOUS EXERCISE, STAND WELL WITH AN ANTEVERTED PELVIS

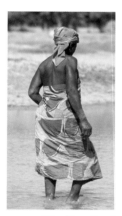

(Burkina Faso)

Be sure your knees are soft, not locked.

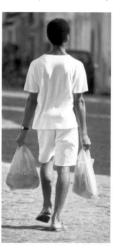

(Brazil)

2 SHIFT YOUR WEIGHT ONTO YOUR LEFT LEG WHILE ENGAGING THE LEFT BUTTOCK MUSCLES. AT THE SAME TIME, BEND YOUR RIGHT KNEE AND HINGE AT THE GROIN

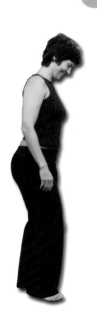

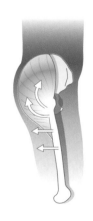

Pause to check for the following:
- Your pelvis remains anteverted.
- Your left thigh bone is pulled back within the flesh of the thigh as your left hamstring contracts. This may be difficult to sense at first.
- There is minimal disturbance in the rest of your body, and your pelvis remains in a horizontal line from left to right.

When initiating a stride, it is helpful to become aware of the action of the buttock muscles to pull the upper part of the femur back within the flesh of the thigh.

HEALTHY MID-STRIDE MUSCLE ACTION

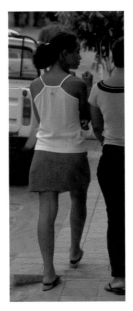

Notice the significant muscle contraction in the left buttock (Brazil)

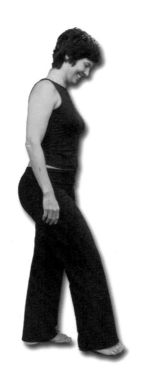

3 EXTEND YOUR RIGHT LEG FORWARD WITHOUT TUCKING THE PELVIS

During this phase, your right leg remains relatively relaxed.

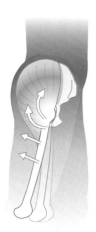

Further contracting the buttock muscles pivots the leg back relative to the torso. Because the foot is firmly positioned on the floor, this action propels the body forward.

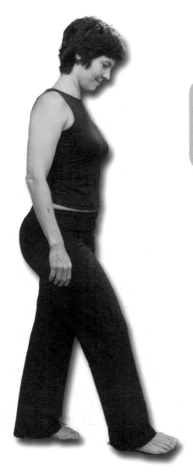

4 AS YOUR RIGHT LEG MOVES FORWARD, INCREASINGLY CONTRACT ALL THE MUSCLES OF YOUR LEFT BUTTOCK TO PROPEL YOU FORWARD

Do not allow the contraction of your buttock muscles to be abrupt, causing a jerky, upward, prancing motion. Rather, make the contraction build gradually to a crescendo, resulting in a controlled forward propulsion.

5 PRESS YOUR LEFT HEEL INTO THE GROUND, KEEP YOUR LEFT LEG STRAIGHT, AND CONTRACT YOUR LEFT GLUTEUS MEDIUS MUSCLE

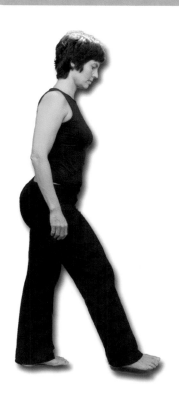

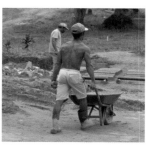

(Brazil)

At the end of the "swing phase" of the right leg, just before your right foot strikes the ground, your left gluteus medius muscle is at its point of maximum contraction. This keeps your weight from falling forward and your right foot from landing with a heavy step.

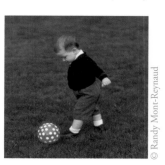

(USA)

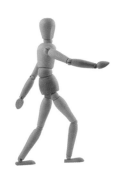

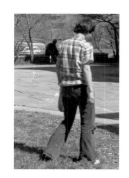

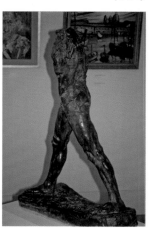

(France)

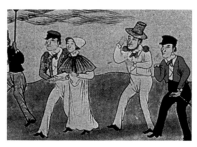

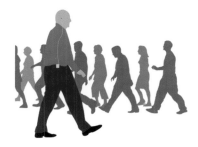

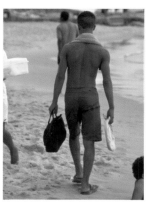

Common mistakes include not contracting the gluteus muscles adequately, contracting the gluteus muscles later than described here, not straightening the back leg, and not leaving the heel on the ground long enough.

(Brazil)

© Randy Mont-Reynaud

EXAMPLES OF LANDING WITH A BENT KNEE IN A HEALTHY STRIDE

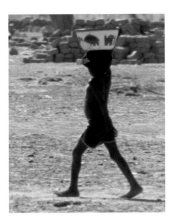

(Burkina Faso)

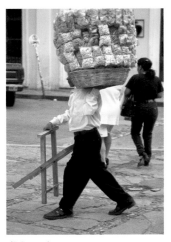

(Mexico)

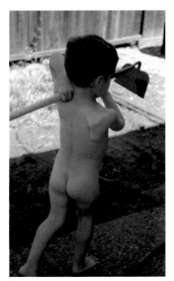

(USA)

6 LOWER YOUR RIGHT FOOT GENTLY TO THE GROUND

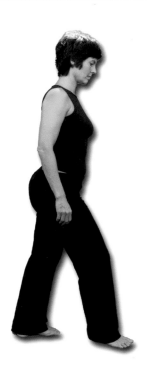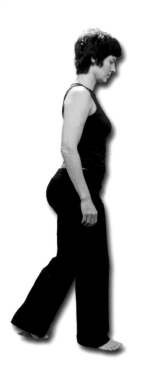

Note that your right heel lands first, but only barely before the rest of the foot. The right knee is slightly bent and soft when your heel touches the ground. After landing, all the buttock muscles of your left leg relax as it becomes the passive leg.

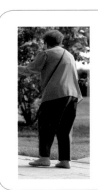

A common mistake is to relax the gluteus medius muscle before the front heel touches the ground. This will result in a heavy step.

7 REPEAT THESE STEPS ON THE OTHER SIDE

Pay particular attention to the muscle contractions in the buttock of the weight-bearing leg.

8 TAKE SEVERAL STEPS WITH A SLOW GAIT, CONCENTRATING ON THE WEIGHT BEARING LEG

GLIDEWALKING: FOCUSING ON THE SWINGING LEG

In a healthy gait, the passive phase is as important as the active phase. Just after the forward foot lands, the muscles in the back leg profoundly relax and the leg drifts forward.

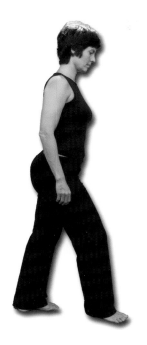

1 STAND AS IF YOU ARE MID-STRIDE

Your left leg is straightened behind you, your left buttock is contracted, and your left heel is pressed into the ground

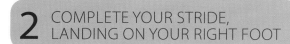

2 COMPLETE YOUR STRIDE, LANDING ON YOUR RIGHT FOOT

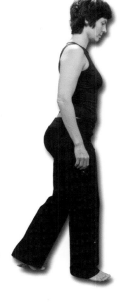

3 CONSCIOUSLY AND COMPLETELY RELAX ALL THE MUSCLES IN THE LEFT HIP AREA, ALLOWING THE LEFT LEG TO DRIFT FORWARD

EXAMPLES OF HEALTHY RELAXATION IN THE BACK LEG AFTER FOOTFALL

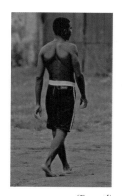

(Brazil)

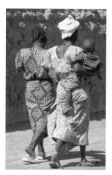

(Burkina Faso)

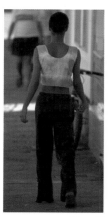

(Brazil)

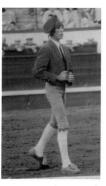

(Portugal)

EXAMPLES OF HEALTHY RELAXATION IN THE SWINGING LEG

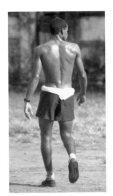

(Brazil)

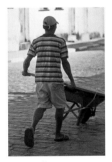

(Brazil)

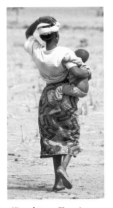

(Burkina Faso)

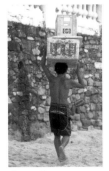

(Brazil)

4 LIFT YOUR LEFT TOE FROM THE GROUND WHILE RETAINING MOST OF THE MUSCLE RELAXATION IN THE HIP JOINT AND ANKLES

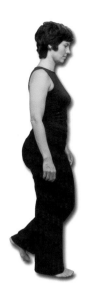

If your ankles are indeed relaxed, someone behind you could see the entire sole of your passive foot. If your hip joint is relaxed, you will feel the pendulum effect.

5 COMPLETE THE STRIDE TO ARRIVE AT THE STARTING POSITION BUT WITH YOUR RIGHT LEG BEHIND YOU

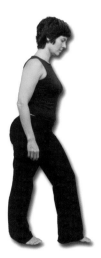

6 TAKE SEVERAL SLOW STEPS, FOCUSING YOUR ATTENTION ON THE SWINGING LEG AND IGNORING THE WEIGHT BEARING LEG

If you find it difficult to relax your muscles quickly following their intense contraction, pause in your stride until it becomes easy.

PUTTING IT ALL TOGETHER: REFINING YOUR GAIT

The active phase contributes power and speed to your gait. The passive phase contributes relaxation and grace. In this section you will combine the phases to walk with strength and grace.

Because this is the most complex lesson in the book, it is easy to feel overwhelmed. Only as you become comfortable with glidewalking should you work to add the refinements in 2 through 5 below.

1 TAKE SEVERAL STEPS, FOCUSING ON BOTH THE ACTIVE AND PASSIVE PHASES IN EACH STRIDE

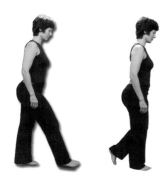

If you find it difficult, as most students do, to alternate between the extreme contraction and extreme relaxation of your muscles, slow your pace.

As with standing, most students feel they are leaning forward when they walk correctly. Resist the urge to "straighten up."

2 PAUSE IN YOUR GAIT JUST AS THE BACK KNEE CROSSES YOUR FRONT KNEE. CHECK YOUR HIP POSITION IN A MIRROR

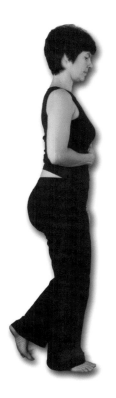

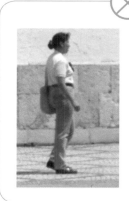

A common mistake is to walk with the pelvis leading, which corrupts the gait. If your pelvis has migrated too far forward, adjust by shifting it backwards.

At this point in the step, your hips should be stacked over the heel of your weight-bearing leg.

AN EXAMPLE OF ACTIVE AND PASSIVE PHASES IN A HEALTHY GAIT

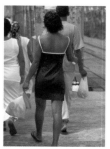

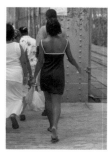

(Brazil)

EXAMPLES OF HEALTHY HIP POSITION MID-STRIDE

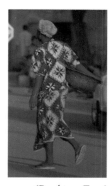

(Burkina Faso)

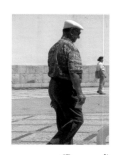

(Portugal)

EXAMPLES OF WALKING ON A LINE

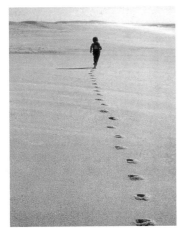

(Portugal)

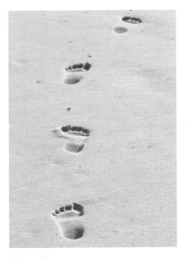

(Brazil)

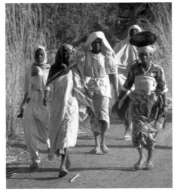

(Burkina Faso)

3 **WALK ON A LINE, WITH THE INNER EDGE OF EACH HEEL TOUCHING THE LINE, AND THE FRONT OF THE FOOT ANGLED SLIGHTLY OUTWARD**

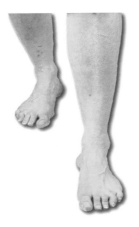

Find a surface with lines, such as a hardwood floor or striated carpet, and straddle one line. Walk in the direction of the line, noticing the orientation of your feet as they contact the floor.
Feel the inner thigh muscles (*adductors*) working to bring the inner heels to this line.

Common mistakes include:

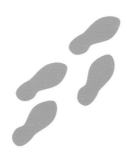

Pointing the toes in

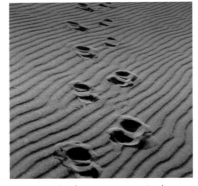

Pointing the feet out excessively

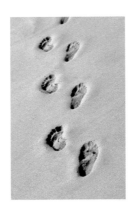

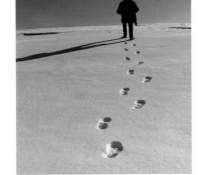

Walking on two lines

4 USE YOUR FEET TO AUGMENT YOUR PUSH-OFF. CONTRACT ALL THE ARCH MUSCLES OF YOUR BACK FOOT SO THAT IT BECOMES A STABLE PLATFORM FOR A POWERFUL PUSH-OFF

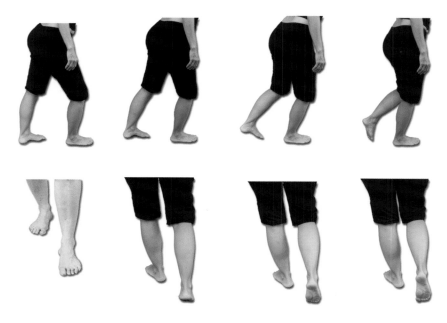

This preserves the shape of your back foot at push-off, when it might otherwise collapse and cause strain to several foot structures.

5 DO A SHOULDER ROLL WITH EACH SHOULDER. THEN PLACE YOUR ARMS BEHIND YOUR BACK WITH ONE HAND CLASPING THE OTHER HAND OR WRIST. TRY TO POSITION THE BACKS OF YOUR WRISTS ON YOUR BUTTOCKS

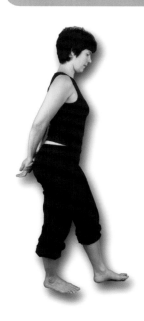

This will help you position your shoulders in a healthy way without having to pay attention to them. It will also help you monitor the action of your buttock muscles.

EXAMPLES OF USING STRONG FOOT ARCH MUSCLES AT PUSH-OFF

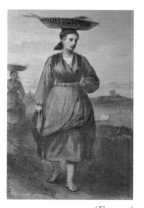

(France)

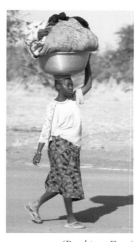

(Burkina Faso)

EXAMPLE OF A HEALTHY SHOULDER POSITION WHILE WALKING

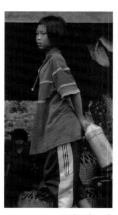

(Thailand)

187

EXAMPLES OF
GLIDEWALKING

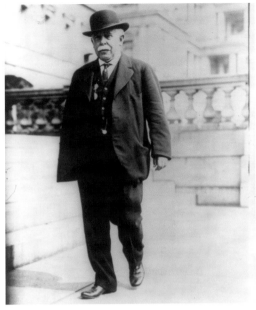

(USA)

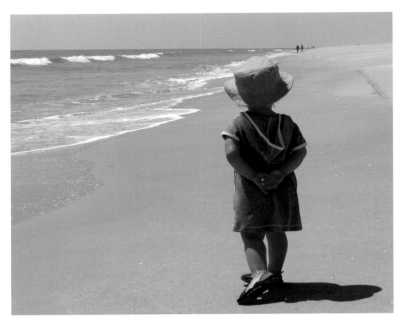

(USA)

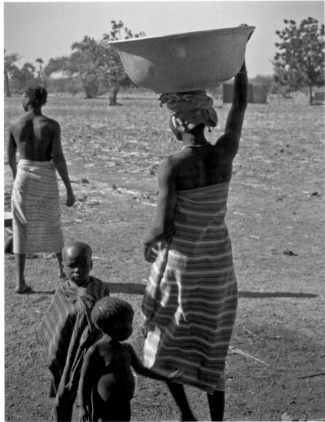

(Burkina Faso)

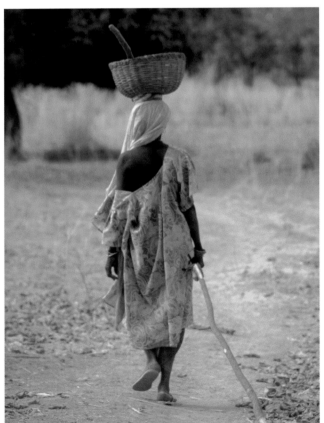

(Burkina Faso)

EXAMPLES OF GLIDEWALKING

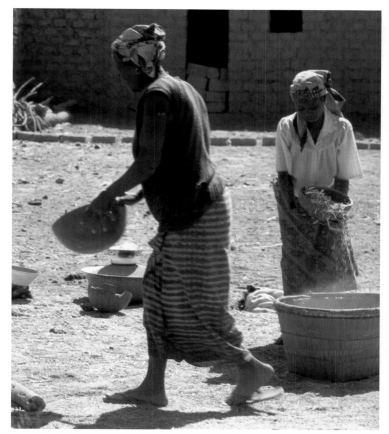

(Burkina Faso)

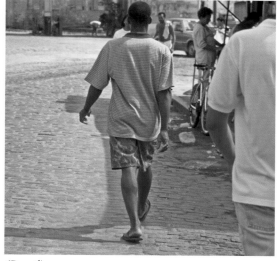

(Brazil)

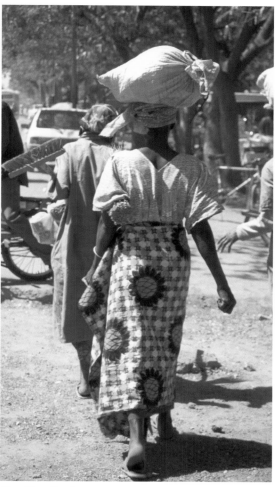

(Burkina Faso)

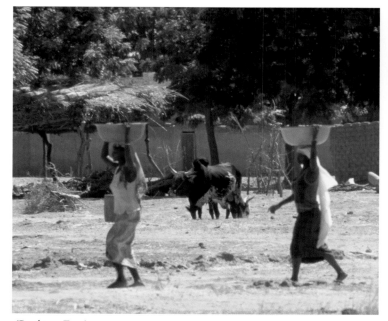

(Burkina Faso)

INDICATIONS OF IMPROVEMENT

Your musculature may change profoundly in the first weeks after learning to glidewalk. Students often report that their buttocks are sore the day after their first walking session. Within a week, they usually may have firmer, higher buttocks. Every step done well is similar to Jane Fonda's "donkey kick" exercise, adding up to a lot of repetitions.

When your walking becomes a series of controlled forward propulsions, your tread is lighter, your movement is more graceful, and your walking experience becomes smoother and calmer. Over time you will strengthen the gluteus, leg, and foot arch muscles and, if you walk briskly, the inner corset. You may notice additional length in your psoas muscle, where before it was tight.

TROUBLESHOOTING

FEELING THAT YOU ARE LEANING FORWARD

As with standing, it is common for students learning this new gait to feel they are leaning forward. To reassure yourself, check in the mirror that from the shoulders to the feet, you are quite upright. (Some people with rigidity in their necks may still have their heads somewhat forward.) In the beginning, intentionally leaning forward just a little can help you discover the right mechanisms in the buttocks and legs.

TENDENCY TO TUCK OR LEAD WIITH THE PELVIS

Even if you understand the concept of leaving your pelvis anteverted throughout your gait, you may find that you have a strong tendency to tuck or lead with the pelvis. Understanding why this is so can help reduce the tendency.

You have probably been using your thigh *(quadriceps)* muscles to advance your front leg and pelvis in your gait. Now you need to use your psoas muscle to advance your front leg and your buttock *(gluteus)* muscles to advance your pelvis. Whereas your quads can work more efficiently when your pelvis is tucked, your psoas and gluteus muscles work more efficiently when your pelvis is anteverted. Changing your pelvic position changes much of the muscle action underlying your gait. This may not be an easy transition.

UNABLE TO COORDINATE BUTTOCK CONTRACTION AND FORWARD THRUST

Become aware of how the buttocks of the back leg contract to propel you forward. Place your hands on your buttocks and sense the contractions as you walk. At this point, the forward thrust may not come solely from your buttock muscles; other muscles may be assisting. Don't worry about it. Over time, as your buttocks strengthen and the sensation of contracting these muscles becomes more familiar, the coordination becomes easier. You will no longer need to use your quadriceps inappropriately to move forward.

DIFFICULTY LEAVING BACK HEEL ON THE FLOOR

To enable the back heel to remain on the floor as long as possible, bend the front knee slightly on landing. It may help to imagine you are walking uphill or skating, or have chewing gum under your back heel. When I teach this aspect of walking, I sometimes walk behind the student and, using my toes, gently hold their heel at the Achilles tendon (fig.8-9). The action may be reminiscent of a sibling stepping on the back of your shoes as you walk.

fig.8-9

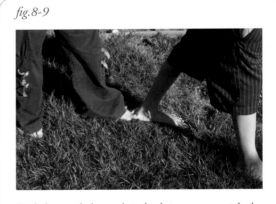

To help people leave their heels in contact with the floor longer than they are used to doing, it helps to step on their heels as they walk.

LOSING TRACK OF YOUR POSTURE

When learning this new gait, students often regress in their overall posture, returning to old patterns. There are so many new things to learn that it's easy to forget good alignment. Pause for a moment to reset your shoulders, your neck and head, and your low back. Be careful not to tuck or lead with the pelvis, or sway the low back in an effort to "straighten up." Look at Troubleshooting in Lesson 6 for reminders on how to align the shoulders and achieve optimal stacking. Tying your arms behind your body (see fig.6-12 on page 143) will help you align your shoulders without having to pay attention to them.

CANNOT COORDINATE ALL THE ELEMENTS OF GLIDEWALKING

For some people it is very difficult to edit their deeply ingrained walking pattern. If you find the material in this chapter too challenging, try an alternative approach: learn and practice the basic Samba step! Chances are, you do not know how to dance the Samba, so you will start with a clean slate, with nothing to unlearn. You can learn the glidewalking motion without the difficulty of unlearning your old gait. This approach works very well.

Learning the Samba

The step taught here is slightly different from the classic three-beat, hip-swinging Samba. This version emphasizes the movements needed for glidewalking (fig.8-10).

1. Take a small step back with the right leg and press the heel into the ground, straightening the right leg and tightening the right buttock muscles. You will need to bend the left (front) knee a little to enable the back heel to reach the floor. This constitutes the first beat.
2. Hold that position for a second beat.
3. Move the right leg forward to return to the starting position.
4. Perform the same motions with the left leg: step back, press the heel into the ground, straighten the leg, and contract the buttock muscle; hold for a beat; return to the starting position.
5. Repeat the movements, alternating the left and right legs, until the movements become familiar.

When you have mastered this movement on both sides and have "memorized" the stance of the back leg, step *forward* into the same stance. Practice this with each leg, going forward and holding each pose for one beat. Next, practice moving forward, alternating steps and smoothing

out the action until it feels like walking. You have just learned the glidewalking motion without the difficulty of unlearning your old gait.

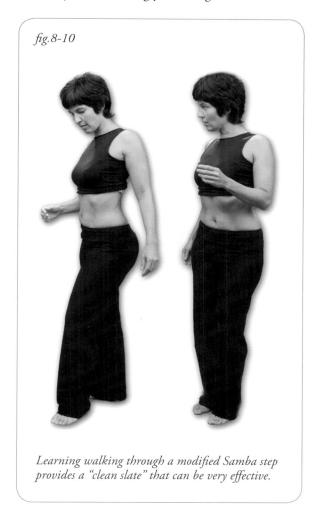

fig.8-10

Learning walking through a modified Samba step provides a "clean slate" that can be very effective.

FURTHER INFORMATION

WALKING ON ONE LINE

The feature of "walking on one line" that you learned in Step 3 on page 186 has an interesting anthropological history. The oldest known human footprints were found in the Olduvai Gorge in northern Tanzania (fig.8-11). They consist of two parallel tracks, thought to belong to an adult and a child who are referred to as the Laetoli duo. Both individuals walked "on a line"; that is to say, the inner heels of each individual touched a single line. This finding has been used as evidence of evolutionary distance between the ancient pair and modern man. The argument, which is correct, is that modern man walks on two lines. But walking on two lines is a very recent cultural distortion in modern industrialized societies. Modern man in more traditional societies elsewhere in the world (as well as in our society in the recent past) walks on one line. The finding that the Laetoli duo walked on a line then becomes an argument not for evolutionary distance, but rather for evolutionary proximity to modern man.

fig.8-11

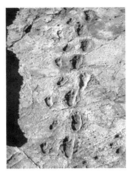

The Laetoli footprints, estimated to date from 3.7 million years ago, show that the bipedal individuals walked "on a line," much as people do today in traditional cultures.

fig.8-12

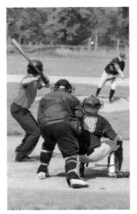 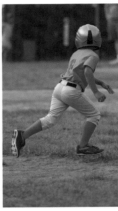

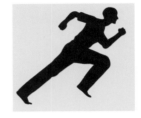

We naturally lean forward when doing demanding activities, as this puts the buttock muscles in a position of mechanical advantage.

GETTING EXTRA POWER IN YOUR STRIDE

Many activities, such as running, hiking uphill, and skating, require extra power in each stride. In these activities we naturally lean forward to put our buttocks in a position of maximum mechanical advantage (fig.8-12). The goal is to use the buttocks in the same way when walking, which is typical in kinesthetically intact cultures. In our culture, when we aren't faced with the added demand of strenuous activity, we tend to tuck the pelvis, which reduces the contribution of the gluteus muscles to our stride.

RUNNING LIKE A KENYAN

If you have observed Kenyan and some other elite runners, you may notice that they run with upright torsos. Their stance may seem to contradict the theory that leaning forward puts your buttocks into a position of mechanical advantage. Most elite runners have healthy curvature in the low back, allowing for both an anteverted pelvis (providing the necessary mechanical advantage to the buttock muscles) and an upright torso. The important factor is the anteverted pelvis, which these runners achieve without leaning forward (fig.8-13).

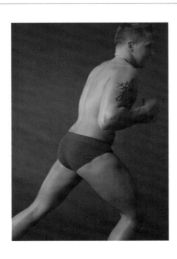

fig.8-13

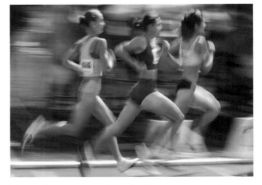

These elite runners show both an anteverted pelvis and an upright torso.

RECAP

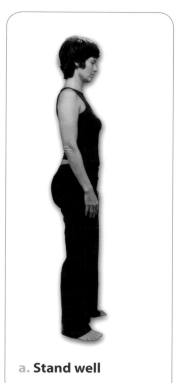

a. Stand well

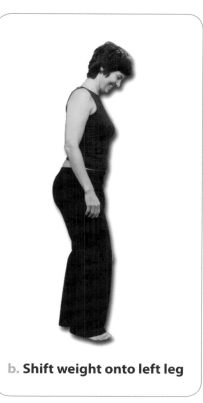

b. Shift weight onto left leg

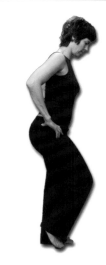

c. Simultaneously:
- **Bend right knee, hinge at hip, let right leg relax**
- **Begin to straighten left leg, tighten left buttock, press left heel into ground**

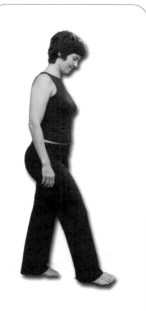

d. Extend right leg forward; increasingly straighten left leg, tighten left buttock

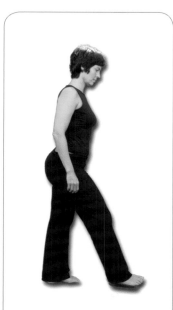

e. Push off strongly with left foot; further straighten left leg, tighten left buttock, press left heel into ground

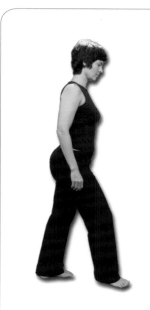

f. Gently place right foot on ground, heel first, knee slightly bent

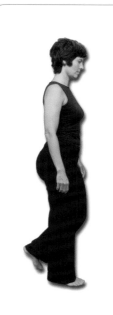

g. Relax left leg

APPENDIX 1
OPTIONAL
EXERCISES

*Strengthening and lengthening key
muscles to accelerate your progress*

One of the special benefits of my method is that it does not require setting aside time for special exercise regimens. However, you may want to perform a few optional exercises early in your training to help you reach a threshold level of strength or flexibility in key muscles. The exercises in this appendix are safe, efficient, and relevant to good posture. Eventually, you will not need them, because as you perform your daily activities with good form, and include appropriate physical exertion in your life, you will meet most of your muscle lengthening and strengthening needs in your everyday life. You will then be in a self-sustaining cycle of healthy posture supporting healthy musculature supporting healthy posture.

When you perform these exercises, especially if your muscles are not warm, be sure to tune in to your body. Do not push yourself to the point of injury or pain.

HOW MUCH AND HOW LONG?

In general, do as much as is comfortable. The exercises should leave you feeling pleasantly fatigued. Many people find it feels right to hold each stretch or pose 30 seconds to a minute. If repetitions are involved, try starting with eight to ten, in two sets.

The exercises are organized into the following categories:

- Strengthening torso muscles

- Strengthening and stretching shoulder muscles

- Strengthening and stretching neck muscles

- Stretching key muscles connecting the torso and legs

- Strengthening key muscles used in walking

EQUIPMENT

You will need the following:
- *A Theraband® or strap*
- *One or two pillows*
- *Rolls made of towels or cotton batting*
- *Hard synthetic balls of various diameters, from 1/2" to 1"*
- *A piece of sturdy fabric about 6' long*
- *A small hand towel or flannel square*
- *A steady object to lean on, such as a desk or counter*
- *A carpeted surface or mat*

STRENGTHENING THE TORSO MUSCLES

Three sets of muscles in your torso warrant your attention. The first, the "rib anchor," holds the front lower edge of the rib cage flush with the abdomen. This maintains the shape of the torso and helps eliminate a sway. The second and third sets of muscles comprise the "inner corset." They lengthen the torso and protect the spine from compression and possible injury. The front part of the inner corset includes the *obliques*, the *upper rectus abdominus*, and the *transversus*. The back part of the inner corset is composed of the deepest layer of back muscles, the *rotatores*.

STRENGTHENING THE ABDOMINAL MUSCLES

The most important exercise for your abdominal muscles should occur throughout the day as they work to maintain the shape and length of your torso. It is *for* performing this function that we want the abdominal muscles to be strong; it is *in* performing this function that the abdominals can become and remain strong. In our society, where many of us engage in sedentary activities for long hours, our abdominal muscles may not be adequately challenged throughout the day. Because they are not kept at a baseline level of strength, the muscles are not up to their task of protecting the spine.

The standard approach for strengthening the abdominals involves exercises such as sit-ups and crunches that distort the spine. Such exercises do strengthen the abdominals, but at the expense of discs and ligaments in the spine. Though there are ways to limit the damage done to the back and neck, it is very difficult to do this, especially for a beginner.

In my approach, the exercises used to strengthen the abdominal muscles would ordinarily distort the spine, if there were no abdominal contraction. You use your abdominal muscles to prevent this distortion and maintain the shape of your spine. In this way you strengthen your abdominals in their natural function of preserving the shape of the spine.

Many exercises for the abdominal muscles are done lying on your back. You will begin by engaging the rib anchor to attain a safe and healthy baseline position.

ENGAGING THE RIB ANCHOR

1. **LENGTHEN YOUR BACK AS YOU LIE DOWN, AS YOU LEARNED TO DO IN LESSON 2**
You will work to preserve the shape of your spine as you do these exercises, but some distortion may occur. Lengthening your back at the start will prevent the distortion from causing problems to your discs. If you do not lengthen your back first and you have some compressed discs, any distortion from the exercises may cause damage.

2. (*OPTIONAL*) **PUT A SMALL TOWEL ROLL, PERHAPS ½ INCH THICK, BETWEEN YOUR LOW BACK AND THE FLOOR. PLACE IT AS LOW AS IT WILL GO WITHOUT LIFTING YOUR BUTTOCKS OR TAILBONE OFF THE FLOOR**
Start by placing the roll in the small of your back where it will fit easily and then pushing the roll down until it won't go any further. This will help support your lumbo-sacral arch (the natural arch low in your back between the last lumbar vertebra and the sacrum), and tip your pelvis forward throughout these exercises.

3. **USE ONE OR MORE PILLOWS UNDER YOUR HEAD AND SHOULDERS. PLACE YOUR ARMS COMFORTABLY AT YOUR SIDES**
When you lie completely flat, the abdominal muscles are close to the end of their range of motion where they are at their weakest. The pillows help to rotate the rib cage forward, putting the abdominal muscles in a position of mechanical advantage. This way you will not strain your neck to achieve a favorable body configuration for working your abdominal muscles.

4. **PRESS THE BACK OF YOUR RIB CAGE AGAINST THE FLOOR WITHOUT LIFTING YOUR "TAIL" OFF THE FLOOR. IT IS EASIEST TO FIND THIS ACTION ON THE EXHALATION. MAINTAIN THE POSITION WHILE CONTINUING TO BREATHE IN AND OUT**
This is a difficult action for many people, but it is important to work toward achieving it. The idea is to isolate the action of the ribcage without tucking the pelvis. Slowing the action down will help you find this isolation. Consider placing your hand under your low back, and feel your ribcage pressing against your hand while leaving the pelvis in its original forward-tipped position.

Now you are ready to proceed with the first set of exercises.

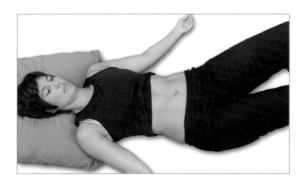
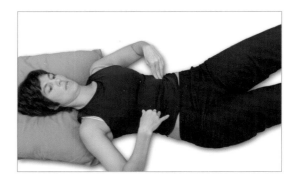

The following is a series of related, increasingly difficult exercises. It's important to master each exercise before progressing to the next.

CYCLING

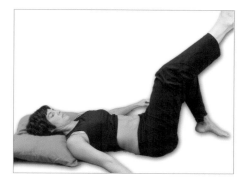

1. FROM THE RIB ANCHOR POSITION, BEND YOUR KNEES AND BRING THEM TO YOUR CHEST

2. STRAIGHTEN YOUR LEGS SO THEY FORM A 90° ANGLE WITH YOUR TORSO

   Be sure to maintain even pressure against the floor with the back of your ribcage. You will find this especially difficult when moving your legs into and out of the starting position above your body. You must use your upper abdominal muscles to anchor your ribcage and prevent your back from swaying.

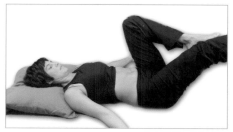

3. WHILE KEEPING THE LOW BACK FLATTENED, ADD THE ACTION OF CYCLING WITH YOUR FEET

4. USE YOUR ABDOMINAL MUSCLES TO STEADY YOUR TORSO

   If your abdominal muscles are lax, your ribcage will lift from the floor, and your torso will tend to squirm from side to side.

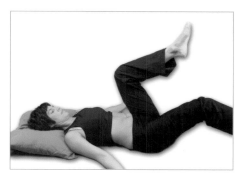

5. WHEN THIS CYCLING EXERCISE FEELS VERY EASY AND YOUR ABDOMINAL MUSCLES ARE READY FOR A GREATER CHALLENGE, MOVE YOUR IMAGINARY BICYCLE PEDALS CLOSER TO THE FLOOR

   With your legs in this position, your abdominal muscles have to work harder to keep the back of your ribcage pressed against the floor. Make sure you do not over-challenge your abdominals. Preserve the shape of the spine throughout the exercise. In this way, your abdominals get a good workout without damaging the discs and ligaments of the spine.

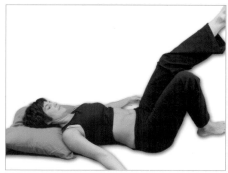

LEG SLIDE

1. FROM THE RIB ANCHOR POSITION, BEND YOUR KNEES AND PLACE YOUR FEET ON THE FLOOR

2. SLOWLY STRAIGHTEN ONE LEG, SLIDING THE FOOT ALONG THE FLOOR
   Keep the weight of the foot light on the floor.

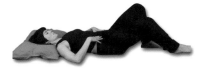 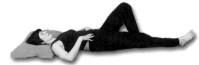

3. WHEN YOUR LEG IS NEARLY STRAIGHT, SLIDE THE FOOT BACK TO ITS STARTING POSITION
   Throughout the range of motion, maintain the pressure of the back of your ribcage against the floor.

4. REPEAT THIS MOTION SEVERAL TIMES AND THEN SWITCH LEGS

5. AS YOUR ABDOMINAL MUSCLES STRENGTHEN, LIGHTEN THE WEIGHT OF YOUR FOOT ON THE FLOOR UNTIL YOUR FOOT IS OFF THE FLOOR

6. WHEN YOUR ABDOMINAL MUSCLES ARE READY FOR EVEN MORE CHALLENGE, DO THE SAME EXERCISE WITH BOTH LEGS AT ONCE

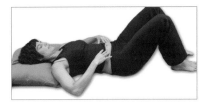

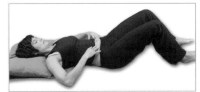

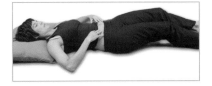

ARM RAISE

1. FROM THE RIB ANCHOR POSITION, RAISE YOUR ARMS TOWARD THE CEILING AND THEN OVER YOUR HEAD
   Be sure to press the back of your ribcage against the floor. The most challenging position is when your arms approach the floor over your head. Raising the arms tends to rotate the ribcage and sway your low back. Your abdominal muscles are challenged to counteract this effect.

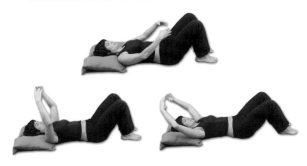

2. LOWER YOUR ARMS BACK TO YOUR SIDES

3. REPEAT THIS MOVEMENT A FEW TIMES
   This exercise also patterns you to reach for things above your head without swaying your back.

4. WHEN YOU ARE FAMILIAR WITH THIS EXERCISE, COMBINE THE LEG SLIDE AND ARM RAISE EXERCISES
   Remember to maintain the shape of your spine while you are moving and stretching all four limbs. This is an excellent exercise for strengthening your core and patterning your muscles.

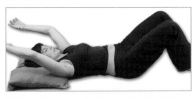

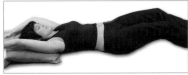

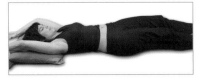

LEG LIFTS

1. FROM THE RIB ANCHOR POSITION, BEND YOUR KNEES AND BRING THEM TO YOUR CHEST

2. STRAIGHTEN YOUR LEGS SO THEY FORM A 90° ANGLE WITH YOUR TORSO

3. LOWER YOUR LEGS TOWARD THE FLOOR WITHOUT MOVING YOUR SPINE
   The challenge here is to keep your spine immobile as your legs travel through their range of motion. If you feel your ribcage begin to lift from the floor, you have gone too far.

4. RETURN YOUR LEGS TO THEIR STARTING POSITION

5. REPEAT THIS MOVEMENT SEVERAL TIMES

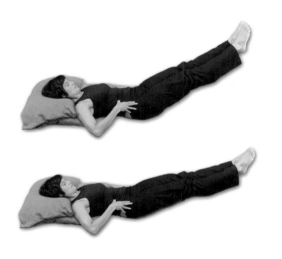

ALPHABET

1. FROM THE RIB ANCHOR POSITION, BEND YOUR KNEES AND BRING THEM TO YOUR CHEST

2. STRAIGHTEN YOUR LEGS SO THEY FORM A 90° ANGLE WITH YOUR TORSO

3. KEEPING YOUR LEGS TOGETHER AND STRAIGHT, USE THEM TO WRITE THE LETTERS OF THE ALPHABET IN THE AIR
   Be sure to keep your ribcage firmly pressed to the floor.

LEG SCISSORS

1. FROM THE RIB ANCHOR POSITION, BEND YOUR KNEES AND BRING THEM TO YOUR CHEST

2. STRAIGHTEN YOUR LEGS SO THEY FORM A 90° ANGLE WITH YOUR TORSO

3. SLICE YOUR LEGS THROUGH THE AIR IN A SIDEWAYS SCISSOR MOVEMENT
   a) Widen your legs.
   b) Bring them together.
   c) Cross one over the other, alternating which leg is on top.

4. FOR A GREATER CHALLENGE, MOVE YOUR LEGS CLOSER TO THE FLOOR
   Again, go only to the point where your abdominals can still press your ribcage firmly to the floor.

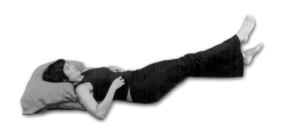

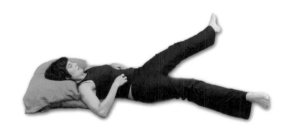

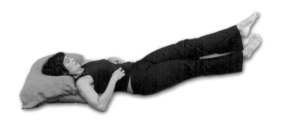

Three yoga poses are particularly effective for strengthening the abdominals: the plank, the side plank, and the boat. Engage your inner corset for extra safety and exercise while doing these poses.

PLANK

1. GET INTO A POSITION ON ALL FOURS, WITH YOUR SHOULDERS DIRECTLY ABOVE YOUR HANDS AND YOUR HIPS DIRECTLY ABOVE YOUR KNEES
   In yoga, this is known as Table Pose.

2. ROLL OPEN YOUR SHOULDERS

3. EXTEND ONE LEG BACK WITH THE TOES CURLED UNDER, THEN EXTEND SECOND LEG
   You are now in push-up position with your arms straight.

4. CHECK YOUR POSITION AND MAKE THE FOLLOWING ADJUSTMENTS AS NECESSARY:
   a. Aim for a straight line from your legs through your torso to your neck.
   b. Resist the tendency to sag or elevate the buttocks out of this line.
   c. Keep the shoulders rolled back and down. Use your muscles to maintain the original relationship between the shoulder blades and the spine.

5. HOLD THIS POSITION UNTIL YOUR MUSCLES FATIGUE
   As you gain strength, you will find you can hold the position longer and longer.

6. REPEAT TWO OR THREE TIMES

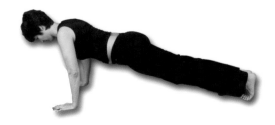

If you find this is too difficult for you, modify your position: Rest your upper body on your forearms rather than your hands, or rest your lower body on your knees rather than your feet.

SIDE PLANK

1. LIE ON YOUR SIDE

2. ROLL YOUR SHOULDERS OPEN AND RAISE YOUR UPPER BODY ONTO YOUR LOWER ARM

3. RAISE YOUR HIPS OFF THE FLOOR SO YOU ARE BALANCING ON YOUR LOWER ARM AND FOOT
   Your body should form a straight line. Don't let the hips sag toward the floor.

4. HOLD THIS POSITION FOR A FEW SECONDS

5. REPEAT ON THE OPPOSITE SIDE

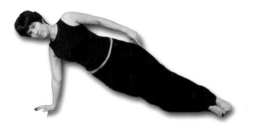

If you find this is too difficult for you, modify your position: Rest your upper body on your forearm rather than your hand, or rest your lower body on your knees rather than your feet.

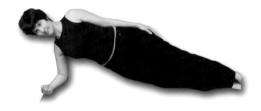

BOAT

1. **SIT ON THE FLOOR, WITH YOUR ARMS BEHIND YOU FOR SUPPORT AND WITH YOUR KNEES BENT**
Be sure your shoulders are rolled back and down, your rib cage is strongly anchored, your inner corset is engaged (see Lesson 5), and your neck is well aligned with the spine.

2. **GRADUALLY LESSEN THE WEIGHT ON YOUR HANDS UNTIL YOU CAN BRING THEM TO YOUR SIDES AND YOUR INNER CORSET FULLY SUPPORTS YOUR BACK**
Be sure to maintain the alignment in the neck and shoulders.

3. **LEAN BACK SLIGHTLY, REDUCING THE WEIGHT ON YOUR FEET, TO FIND A NATURAL BALANCE POINT**
As you do this, work to maintain the original alignment throughout your torso.

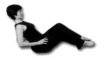

4. **LIFT YOUR FEET FROM THE FLOOR WITH BENT KNEES**
Be sure you don't tuck your pelvis as you lift your feet.

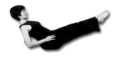

5. **IF POSSIBLE, STRAIGHTEN YOUR LEGS**
Again, be sure to hold your torso steady.

6. **HOLD THIS POSITION UNTIL MUSCLE FATIGUE**

7. **REPEAT TWO OR THREE TIMES**

SAMBA

Another very effective – and fun – way to strengthen your abdominal muscles is to practice the Samba. Refer to page 191 in Lesson 8 to learn the basic dance steps. Then consider taking a class or renting an instructional video. You will learn to move your hips a great deal, motored by action in the legs, while your upper torso remains still or moves with a separate action. Isolating the actions of the upper and lower body challenges the abdominal muscles in complex and constantly changing ways. If you engage your inner corset to lengthen your torso as you twist and undulate, your abdominal muscles will get an even more intense workout.

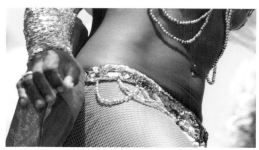

(Brazil)

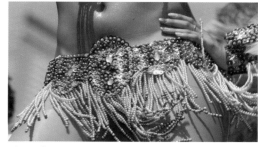

(Brazil)

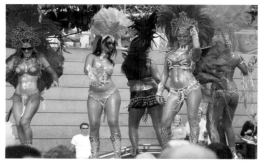

(Norway)

203

STRENGTHENING THE DEEP MUSCLES OF THE BACK

When you engage your inner corset, you contract the deep muscles of the back bilaterally (both sides at once). The exercises in this section are particularly effective at isolating these muscles, one side at a time, to strengthen them.

OPPOSITE ARM/LEG STRETCH

1. **BEGIN ON ALL FOURS, WITH YOUR HANDS BENEATH YOUR SHOULDERS AND YOUR KNEES BENEATH YOUR HIPS**
   Engage your abdominal muscles so that your back does not sway. Allow your pelvis to tip forward comfortably. Be sure that your shoulders remain rolled back.

2. **STRAIGHTEN YOUR RIGHT ARM OUT IN FRONT OF YOU AS YOU LIFT AND STRAIGHTEN YOUR LEFT LEG BEHIND YOU. HOLD FOR A FEW SECONDS**
   Maintain your torso position throughout this movement.

3. **REPEAT WITH THE OPPOSITE ARM AND LEG**

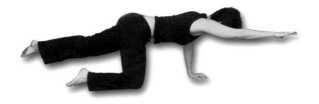

WARRIOR III

1. **BEGIN IN A COMFORTABLE STANDING POSITION**
   Be sure your feet are in kidney-bean shape and your legs are externally rotated. This will enable your pelvis to settle well in Step 2.

2. **KEEPING THE HIPS SQUARE, HINGE FORWARD AT THE HIPS AS YOU LIFT YOUR LEFT LEG STRAIGHT BEHIND YOU**
   Do not sway your back. Use your *gluteus medius* muscles, not your back, to raise the leg. Use the abdominals to prevent any distortion in the torso.

3. **WHEN YOU ARE BALANCED IN THIS POSITION, RAISE YOUR ARMS OVER YOUR HEAD SO THEY FORM A STRAIGHT LINE WITH YOUR TORSO AND RAISED LEG**
   Your body forms an extended T shape, balanced on the left leg. Bend the left leg to help maintain balance. If necessary, perform this exercise beside a wall or chair that you can use for balance.

4. **HOLD THIS POSITION FOR A FEW SECONDS**

5. **REPEAT WITH THE RIGHT LEG ON THE OTHER SIDE**

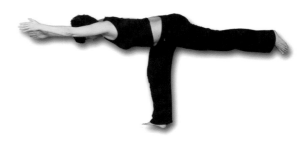

STRENGTHENING AND STRETCHING THE MUSCLES IN THE SHOULDER AREA

To settle the shoulders in a healthy position requires relaxed pectoral and trapezius muscles, and toned rhomboid muscles. All these muscles affect shoulder and arm posture, which influences how the spine stacks. Relaxed pectoral muscles allow the chest cavity to expand freely, facilitating deep inhalation. Relaxed trapezius muscles allow a healthy spacing in the upper thoracic and cervical spine. Relaxed pectoral and trapezius muscles permit the arms to move independently of the torso. Strong rhomboid muscles help peg the shoulders down and back along the torso.

For some people, occasional shoulder rolls may be enough to return the shoulders to a good baseline position. For others, one or more of the following exercises may be helpful.

PEC STRETCH

Begin by positioning yourself well, tallstanding or stacksitting. For all of these exercises, maintaining a good baseline position is important to protect your muscles and joints.

VARIATION 1

1. BEGIN BY PERFORMING A SHOULDER ROLL
   If you start with your shoulders in a healthy position, that position becomes locked into place during this exercise.

2. INTERLACE THE FINGERS BEHIND THE BACK WITH PALMS FACING EACH OTHER

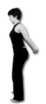

3. ANCHOR THE RIBCAGE
   Contract the upper abdominal muscles to prevent a sway in your back.

4. MOVE THE SHOULDERS FURTHER BACK AND DOWN. ACTIVELY LENGTHEN THE BACK OF YOUR NECK WITH YOUR CHIN ANGLED DOWN WHILE DOING THIS

5. STRAIGHTEN AND RAISE THE ARMS
   Be sure to stop short of distorting your torso or straining your neck or upper shoulders.

6. HOLD FOR A FEW SECONDS

VARIATION 2

In Step 2 above, with fingers interlaced, try rotating palms inward and downward. Continue with the remaining steps.

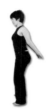

VARIATION 3

In Step 2 above, with fingers interlaced, try rotating palms outward and downward. Continue with the remaining steps.

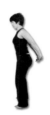

VARIATION 4

1. BEGIN BY PERFORMING A SHOULDER ROLL

2. WRAP A STRAP OR THERABAND® BEHIND THE BACK AND HOLD ONE END IN EACH HAND
   Hold each end so that the band lies along the inner forearm and your palms face up.

3. ATTEMPT TO LIFT THE BAND BACK AWAY FROM YOUR SPINE BY MOVING YOUR ARMS OUT AND BACK
   Be sure to anchor the rib cage, avoiding a sway, and maintain length in the back of the neck.

4. HOLD THE POSITION FOR 30 SECONDS

5. REPEAT SEVERAL TIMES

RHOMBOID TONER

1. BEGIN BY PERFORMING A SHOULDER ROLL
   It's important to begin with a healthy shoulder position to place the rhomboids in a position of mechanical advantage.

2. PIN ELBOWS TO YOUR SIDES AND BEND YOUR ELBOWS TO A 90° ANGLE IN THE FRONT
   The position is similar to when you're carrying a tray.

3. GRAB A THERABAND® OR STRAP
   Be sure not to distort the wrists; keep them firm to avoid unnecessary strain.

4. PRESSING YOUR ELBOWS AGAINST YOUR SIDES, DRAW YOUR SHOULDER BLADES AS CLOSE TOGETHER AS YOU CAN
   Naturally your hands will move away from each other. The band or strap provides resistance to this motion, challenging the rhomboids.

   Be sure not to tense the shoulders or neck.

5. HOLD FOR A FEW SECONDS

TRAP STRETCH

Caution: **If you have neck problems (herniated discs or bone spurs), skip this exercise.**

1. BEGIN BY PERFORMING A SHOULDER ROLL
   Be sure to begin with a healthy shoulder position so that the exercise targets the most relevant part of the trapezius muscle.

2. PLACE THE PALM OF YOUR RIGHT HAND OVER YOUR HEAD NEAR YOUR LEFT EAR

3. USE YOUR HAND TO LENGTHEN YOUR NECK AS YOU GENTLY ALLOW THE WEIGHT OF YOUR RIGHT ARM TO PULL YOUR HEAD CLOSER TO YOUR RIGHT SHOULDER
   Do not force this movement.

4. GENTLY PRESS THE HEEL OF YOUR LEFT HAND DOWN TO AUGMENT THE STRETCH

5. HOLD THIS POSITION FOR A FEW SECONDS

6. REPEAT ON THE OTHER SIDE

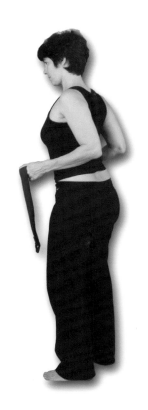

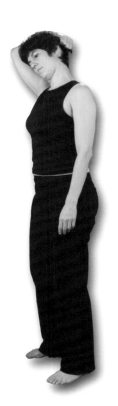

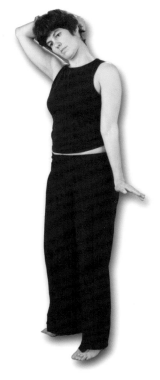

STRENGTHENING THE NECK MUSCLES

1. FOLD A 6-FOOT LENGTH OF FABRIC INTO A 6-INCH WIDE BAND

2. WRAP THE FABRIC BAND BEHIND THE NECK AND HOLD ONE END IN EACH HAND

3. GET INTO A POSITION ON ALL FOURS, WITH YOUR SHOULDERS DIRECTLY ABOVE YOUR HANDS AND YOUR HIPS DIRECTLY ABOVE YOUR KNEES

4. ANCHOR THE FABRIC BAND SECURELY UNDER YOUR HANDS
   Be sure the band is snug against the back of the neck.

5. USE YOUR NECK MUSCLES TO PULL BACK (UP) AGAINST THE BAND

6. HOLD FOR 10 SECONDS

7. REPEAT SEVERAL TIMES

STRETCHING THE NECK MUSCLES

1. BEGIN BY POSITIONING YOURSELF WELL, TALLSTANDING OR STACKSITTING (a)

2. TRANSLATE YOUR FACE FORWARD TILL YOU FEEL A SIGNIFICANT STRETCH IN YOUR NECK MUSCLES (b, c)
   Your face remains in the same orientation to the ground throughout the stretch.

3. HOLD THE STRETCH FOR A FEW SECONDS

4. SHIFT YOUR FACE BACKWARDS BEYOND WHERE YOU WERE AT THE START OF THE EXERCISE (d)
   You will feel a stretch as you lengthen the back of your neck.

5. AUGMENT THE STRETCH BY PULLING BACKWARDS AND UPWARDS ON THE HAIR AT THE BASE OF YOUR SKULL

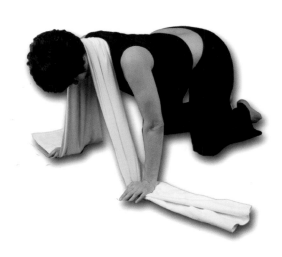

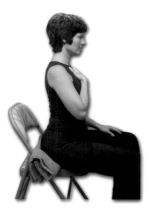

a.

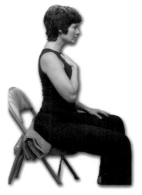

b.

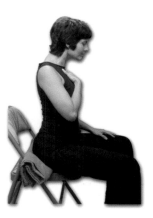

c.

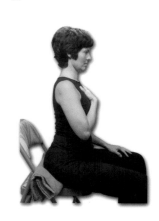

d.

STRETCHING THE KEY MUSCLES THAT CONNECT THE TORSO AND LEGS

Ideally, your legs are able to move independently of your torso. This requires flexibility in several muscles, such as the hamstrings, psoas, and external hip rotators. Length in the hamstring muscles is essential to a healthy pelvic position and healthy bending. A lengthened psoas, one of the key muscles in the groin, facilitates good alignment in the lumbar spine and a healthy stride. Flexible external hip rotator muscles permit the pelvis to form an acute angle with the leg bones for deep bending.

STRETCHING THE HAMSTRINGS

These two stretches are safe and effective for lengthening the hamstring muscles. The hamstrings attach to the sitz bones, and tight hamstrings force the pelvis into a tuck (*retroversion*). If you have short hamstrings, lengthening them is vital to the success of your posture work.

WALL STRETCH

1. STAND WELL, ABOUT TWO TO THREE FEET FROM AND FACING A WALL
   The distance depends on your hamstring flexibility and the length of your upper body. You may need to adjust your position.

2. HINGE AT YOUR HIPS AS YOU PLACE YOUR HANDS ON THE WALL

3. LEAVE HANDS ON WALL ABOVE HEAD
   This lets your shoulders stretch backwards.

4. IF YOU CAN BEND FURTHER, LET YOUR TORSO MOVE TOWARD THE FLOOR AS FAR AS THE HAMSTRINGS WILL TOLERATE
   This will increase your shoulder stretch. If it is too intense, let your hands slide down the wall as you move your torso.

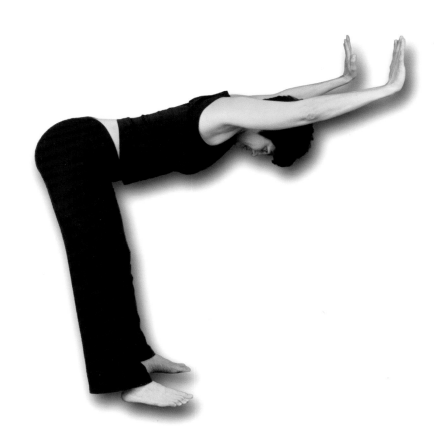

LYING HAMSTRING STRETCH

1. LENGTHEN YOUR BACK AS YOU LIE DOWN, AS YOU LEARNED TO DO IN LESSON 2

2. PLACE A PILLOW UNDER YOUR HEAD AND SHOULDERS, IF THAT MAKES YOU MORE COMFORTABLE

3. HOLDING ONE END OF A STRAP IN EACH HAND, LOOP THE STRAP AROUND THE BALL OF YOUR RIGHT FOOT, AND THEN STRAIGHTEN YOUR LEG (a)
   You may also bend your leg slightly throughout this exercise.

   Keep your arms outstretched and your shoulder blades fixed in position. Don't allow your shoulders to pull forward.

4. LIFT YOUR RIGHT LEG UPWARD TOWARD YOUR HEAD UNTIL YOU FEEL A SIGNIFICANT HAMSTRING STRETCH
   Do not overstretch.

5. HOLD BOTH STRAP ENDS WITH THE RIGHT HAND

6. GENTLY ALLOW THE LEG TO MOVE TO THE RIGHT, TOWARD THE FLOOR, WITHOUT RAISING YOUR LEFT HIP FROM THE FLOOR (b)
   If it helps, use your left hand to hold your left hip to the floor.

7. MOVE YOUR RIGHT LEG BACK UPWARD

8. SWITCH THE STRAP ENDS TO THE LEFT HAND

9. ALLOW YOUR LEG TO FALL GENTLY TO THE LEFT, ACROSS YOUR BODY, TOWARD THE FLOOR (c)
   Do not let your right hip lift from the floor. Your leg will probably not travel very far from vertical.

10. REPEAT THESE STEPS WITH THE LEFT LEG (d,e,f)

a.

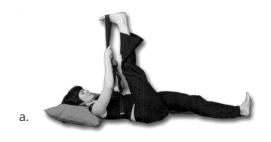

b.

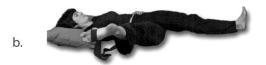

c.

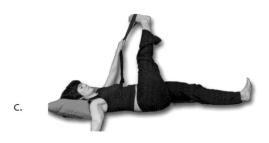

d.

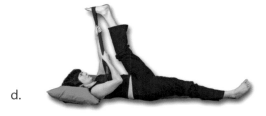

e.

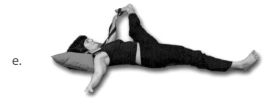

f.

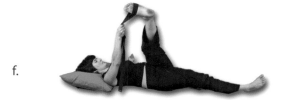

STRETCHING THE EXTERNAL HIP ROTATOR MUSCLES

PAPER CLIP

1. LENGTHEN YOUR BACK AS YOU LIE DOWN, AS YOU LEARNED TO DO IN LESSON 2

2. PLACE A PILLOW UNDER YOUR HEAD AND SHOULDERS IF IT MAKES YOU MORE COMFORTABLE

3. BEND BOTH KNEES AND PLACE YOUR FEET ON THE FLOOR

4. PLACE THE RIGHT ANKLE ACROSS THE LEFT KNEE

5. INTERLACE YOUR FINGERS EITHER BEHIND YOUR LEFT THIGH OR AROUND YOUR LEFT SHIN, LIFTING YOUR LEFT FOOT OFF THE FLOOR (a)
You can use a strap to prevent any distortion in your shoulders or torso (b).

6. DRAW BOTH LEGS TOWARD YOUR CHEST UNTIL YOU SENSE A SIGNIFICANT STRETCH
Again, do not stretch to the point of discomfort.

7. LOWER THE LEGS UNTIL YOUR LEFT FOOT IS ON THE FLOOR; THEN RELEASE

8. REPEAT ON THE OTHER SIDE (c) (d)

LENGTHENING THE PSOAS MUSCLES

LUNGE

1. STAND WELL WITH YOUR FEET ABOUT HIP-WIDTH APART

2. BEND FORWARD WITH A STRAIGHT BACK, PLACING YOUR HANDS TO THE FLOOR OUTSIDE YOUR FEET OR RESTING ON YOUR KNEES
Bend your knees as necessary.

3. EXTEND ONE LEG FAR BACK, OPTIONALLY RESTING THE KNEE ON THE GROUND
Keep the hips square to the ground. Be sure the forward knee does not bend more than 90° or extend in front of the ankle.

4. LET THE PELVIS SINK TOWARD THE FLOOR
This results in a strong stretch in the groin.

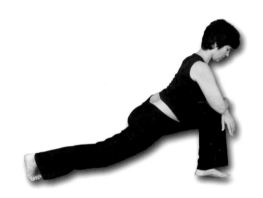

5. REPEAT ON THE OTHER SIDE

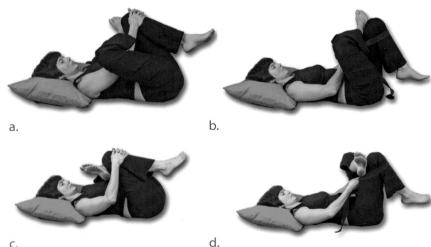

a.

b.

c.

d.

STRENGTHENING KEY MUSCLES USED IN WALKING

Strong arch muscles are essential to the health of the foot and protect foot ligaments from being overstretched. These muscles contribute to a strong push-off when walking. The gluteus medius muscles of the buttocks help give you a healthy gait with a soft landing, contribute to pelvic anteversion, and help externally rotate your legs. The tibialis anterior muscles help you create and support a kidney-bean shape in your feet and help externally rotate your knees.

STRENGTHENING THE ARCH MUSCLES

Achieving a kidney-bean shape in your foot substantially restores the inner arch, the most important of the three arches of the foot. The following exercises further strengthen it, as well as the outer and transverse arches.

INCH WORM

1. WHILE STANDING OR SITTING WELL, PLACE YOUR FEET INTO KIDNEY-BEAN SHAPE

2. RELEASE MOST OF THE WEIGHT FROM ONE FOOT

3. FIX THE TOES OF THE UNWEIGHTED TO THE FLOOR AND CONTRACT ALL THE ARCH MUSCLES IN THE BOTTOM OF THE FOOT (a)
   Your objective is to shorten the foot into an arched shape, drawing the heel closer to the toes.

4. FIX THE HEEL TO THE FLOOR, RELEASE THE TOES AND RELAX ALL THE ARCH MUSCLES
   Allow your foot to return to its longer length.

5. REACH FORWARD WITH THE TOES AND FIX THEM TO THE FLOOR IN THIS NEW POSITION (b)
   Your toes should be slightly ahead of their starting position; they have "inched" forward.

6. REPEAT STEPS 1 - 4 SEVERAL TIMES (c, d) UNTIL YOUR FOOT HAS CREPT ABOUT 6 INCHES FORWARD

7. FIX THE HEEL TO THE FLOOR
   You will now reverse the action to move your foot backwards.

8. RELEASE THE TOES FROM THE FLOOR WHILE CONTRACTING THE ARCH MUSCLES (e)
   The toes draw back toward the heel and the foot shortens.

9. FIX THE TOES TO THE FLOOR AND RELEASE THE CONTRACTION OF THE ARCH MUSCLES (f)
   This allows the heel to move backwards.

10. REPEAT STEPS 7 – 9 SEVERAL TIMES UNTIL YOUR FOOT RETURNS TO ITS STARTING POSITION (g,h)
    It is common for beginners to contract their toes more than their arches. Try to maximize the contraction of your arches while minimizing the contraction of your toes. Over time you will improve your ability to isolate these movements.

11. REPEAT THIS COMPLETE SERIES WITH THE OTHER FOOT

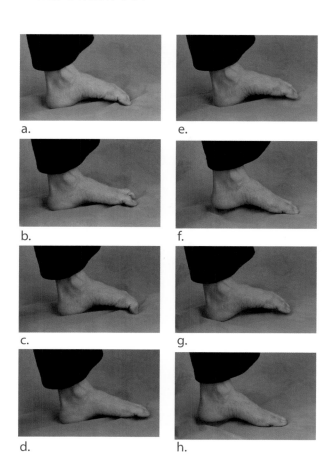

a.
e.
b.
f.
c.
g.
d.
h.

EAT THE CLOTH

1. SPREAD A HAND TOWEL OR SMALL CLOTH ON THE FLOOR
   Use a cloth with some texture, such as terry cloth. Avoid slippery fabrics like silk.

2. WHILE STANDING OR SITTING WELL, PLACE ONE FOOT ON THE EDGE OF THE CLOTH CLOSEST TO YOU (a)

3. USING JUST YOUR FOOT, TRY TO GATHER THE CLOTH UNDER THE FOOT (b)
   This exercise strengthens the muscles that control the underside of your foot.

4. REPEAT WITH THE OTHER FOOT

GRAB THE BALL

1. PLACE A SMALL BALL ON THE FLOOR
   It is useful to have various sized superballs for this exercise. Most students begin with a ball of one-half to one inch in diameter.

2. WHILE STANDING OR SITTING WELL, TRY TO GRAB THE BALL WITH ONE FOOT
   Initially, you may only be able to grab a ball with your toes. Work to grab increasingly larger balls. As your arches grow stronger, you may be able to grab a ball under your transverse arch.

3. REPEAT THESE STEPS WITH THE OTHER FOOT

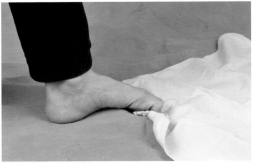

a.

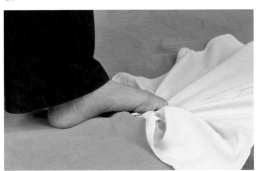

b.

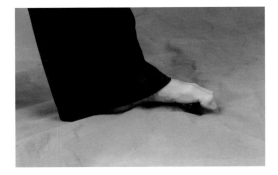

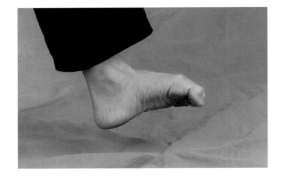

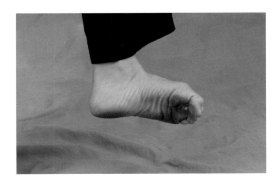

STRENGTHENING THE GLUTEUS MEDIUS MUSCLES

In this exercise, as you lift your leg, you obviously strengthen the gluteus medius muscle on that side. However, you also exercise the same muscle on the other side as it works to maintain a level pelvis.

1. STAND WITH SOFT KNEES AND KIDNEY-BEAN SHAPED FEET

2. SHIFT YOUR WEIGHT TO YOUR LEFT FOOT
   Try to minimize any disturbance to the rest of your body.

3. ROTATE THE RIGHT LEG OUTWARD AT THE HIP, PIVOTING YOUR HEEL (a)
   The toes of your right foot are now pointing to the side. This outward rotation isolates the gluteus medius muscle of your right leg.

4. BEND YOUR RIGHT KNEE AND RAISE THE LEG BACKWARDS (b)
   Be aware that you are engaging your gluteal muscles. Leave the pelvis in its original position as you raise your leg.

5. PLACE YOUR LEFT HAND ON YOUR LOW BACK TO ENSURE YOU KEEP THIS AREA STEADY AS YOU LIFT YOUR LEG (c)
   Use your abdominal muscles to keep your back steady.

6. BEND YOUR BODY FORWARD TO RAISE YOUR LEG HIGHER, HINGING AT THE GROIN (d)
   If necessary, steady yourself by holding onto a chair or wall. As you balance yourself without leaning too heavily on the support, you also exercise your left gluteus medius muscle. With practice you may no longer need to use a support (e, f)

7. LOWER YOUR LEG A LITTLE AND RAISE IT AGAIN

8. REPEAT THESE STEPS ON THE OPPOSITE SIDE
   Repeat this motion in sets of 20 (or a number of your choice). It is helpful to do this to the beat of music you enjoy.

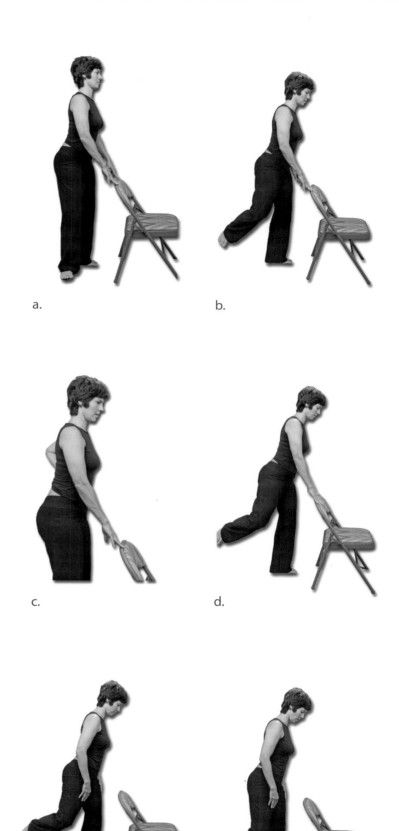

a.

b.

c.

d.

e.

f.

STRENGTHENING THE TIBIALIS ANTERIOR

This muscle enables you to create and maintain a kidney-bean shape in your foot. It is also the muscle associated with shin splints and fallen arches. When the muscle is weak and you place demands on it, as in running and long-distance walking, it can cause significant pain. The following exercise, which you might want to do to music with a driving beat, strengthens the muscle very efficiently.

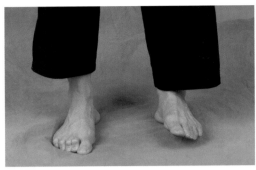

a.

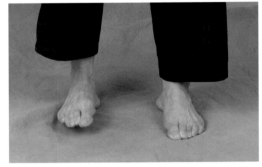

b.

1. STAND WITH SOFT KNEES AND KIDNEY-BEAN SHAPED FEET
   Engage all the arch muscles of the foot to emphasize its convex shape.

2. SHIFT ALL YOUR WEIGHT ONTO YOUR HEELS
   Allow your body to hinge forward slightly at the hip joint to maintain your balance.

3. WHILE MAINTAINING YOUR FOOT SHAPE, LIFT THE FRONT OF ONE FOOT OFF THE FLOOR (a)
   Be sure not to curl your toes upward as you do this.

4. REPLACE THAT FOOT TO THE FLOOR AS YOU LIFT THE OTHER FOOT (b)
   Notice that your entire weight remains on your heels.

5. REPEAT THE MOVEMENT, INCREASING THE SPEED UNTIL YOU FEEL MUSCLE FATIGUE

6. ALLOW YOUR MUSCLES TO RECOVER. THEN REPEAT THE EXERCISE

TROUBLESHOOTING

STIFFNESS OR PAIN

You may experience some soreness or stiffness in the days following these exercises. This is completely normal when you exercise muscles that are out of shape. However, if you experience significant pain during or after performing any of these exercises, you may be stretching or strengthening too vigorously. Let your body recover for a day or two. Then proceed, building up more slowly in intensity and repetitions.

LACK OF IMPROVEMENT

Many of these exercises help you create additional length in your muscles. However, maintaining the new length requires that you use the lengthened muscles in your everyday stance and activities. Brief minutes spent performing targeted exercises may not be sufficient to overcome hours of poor posture. The combination of working on your posture and performing relevant exercises is the fastest way of making change.

FAILURE TO EXERCISE

Some of you will have trouble finding time to perform even a few targeted exercises. If you simply cannot work them into your routine, don't worry about it! If you perform your everyday activities with increased awareness and improved form, you will still make good progress.

FURTHER INFORMATION

Of the countless exercises and regimens available today, many have relatively little value, and some can even cause damage. For example, traditional back extension exercises strengthen the *erector spinae* muscles. However, often the problem with these muscles is that they are too tight, not too weak. In this case, performing back extensions may exacerbate the real problem.

Similarly, traditional crunches target the *rectus abdominus* muscle, can put strain on the lumbar and cervical discs and ligaments, potentially causing serious damage.

People often ask me about the value of the exercise circuits at gyms and fitness centers. In a society where some people interface with little more than their computer all day long, a gym can provide valuable human interaction. Weight machines target specific muscles and track specific actions, thus adequately challenging major muscle groups safely. In addition, users benefit from feedback on their strength and progress. However, because circuit machines control your actions, they do not provide the opportunity for the mixed movements of everyday activities. It is best to mix any exercise regimen with a variety of physical activities.

APPENDIX 2
ANATOMY

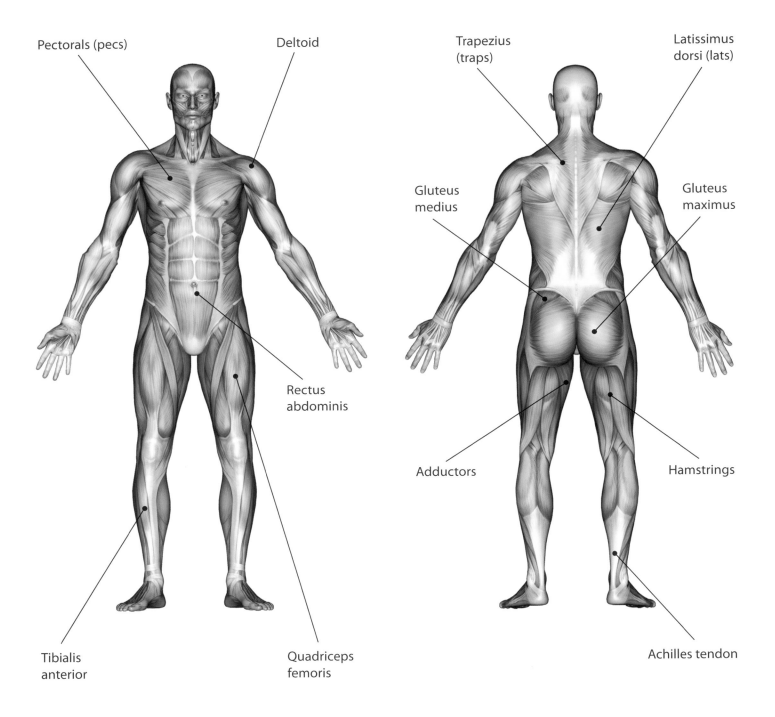

Pectorals (pecs)

Deltoid

Trapezius (traps)

Latissimus dorsi (lats)

Gluteus medius

Gluteus maximus

Rectus abdominis

Adductors

Hamstrings

Tibialis anterior

Quadriceps femoris

Achilles tendon

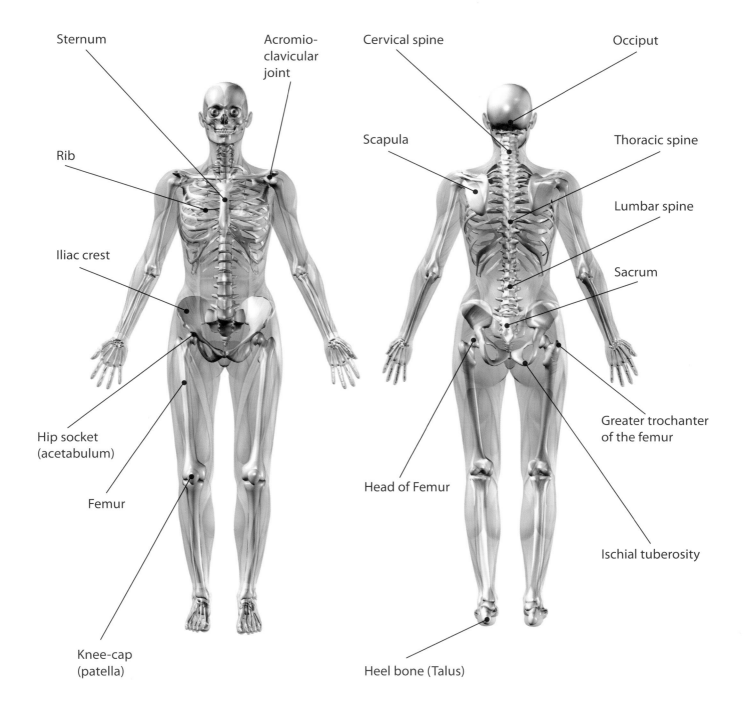

Sternum

Acromio-clavicular joint

Cervical spine

Occiput

Rib

Scapula

Thoracic spine

Lumbar spine

Iliac crest

Sacrum

Hip socket (acetabulum)

Greater trochanter of the femur

Femur

Head of Femur

Ischial tuberosity

Knee-cap (patella)

Heel bone (Talus)

GLOSSARY

ABDOMINAL OBLIQUE MUSCLES
See Oblique muscles.

ACETABULUM
The socket of the hip bone (ox coxa) into which the head of the femur fits.

ACHILLES TENDON
The tendon of the gastrocnemius (large muscle on the posterior of the leg) and soleus (broad, flat calf muscle).

ARCHES OF THE FOOT: INNER, OUTER, AND TRANSVERSE
The inner or medial longitudinal arch runs on the inside of the foot. The outer or lateral longitudinal arch runs along the outside of the foot. The transverse or metatarsal arch runs across the ball of the foot.

ACROMIOCLAVICULAR JOINT
The joint between the clavicle (the long bone of the shoulder girdle running between the sternum and the shoulder blade) and the scapula (the shoulder blade).

ANTEVERSION
Inclining forward without bending (cf. retroversion).

BACKBONE
The set of vertebrae that extends from the cranium to the coccyx, and provides support and a flexible bony case for the spinal cord. The backbone is composed of 33 vertebrae (7 cervical, 12 thoracic, 5 lumbar, 5 fused sacral – forming the sacrum, 4 fused coccygeal – forming the coccyx).

BODY SCAN
A conscious and systematic focusing of one's attention on each part of the body. One method is to begin with the toes and feet, move upward through the legs and torso to the shoulders, then down the arms to the hands and fingers. Last, scan the neck and head.

CERVICAL SPINE
The neck portion of the spine, composed of the first seven vertebra (C1-C7) (cf. thoracic spine, lumbar spine).

CLAVICLE, OR COLLAR BONE
A doubly-curved long bone that connects the arm to the body. It is located directly above the first rib.

DOWAGER'S HUMP
An extreme forward bending or curving of the spine.

ELECTRO-MYELOGRAPHY
A method of recording the electrical currents generated in an active muscle.

ERECTOR SPINAE MUSCLE (SACROSPINALIS)
A large muscle of the back that supports the spinal column and head.

EXTERNAL ROTATION (OF THE HIP)
The process of turning the leg outward at the hip joint, so the legs and feet are not parallel, but splayed with the heels closer together than the toes.

FEMUR
The large bone of the thigh extending from the hip to the knee; the longest and strongest bone of the skeleton.

GLUTEUS MEDIUS MUSCLE
One of three major muscles of the buttocks (the gluteus maximus, gluteus medius, and gluteus minimus). Located in the upper, outer quadrant of buttock, the gluteus medius moves the leg to the side and rotates the thigh.

HAMSTRING MUSCLES
The group of three muscles at the back of the thigh.

ILIAC CREST
The upper, outer free edge of the ilium (a pelvic bone)

INTERNAL CORSET
The collection of muscles between the ribs and hips that help lengthen and support the spine.

ISCHIAL TUBEROSITIES
The rounded portion of the lower hip bones (ischia); also called sitz bones.

KIDNEY-BEAN SHAPED FEET
The healthy shape of the feet with the heels pivoted inward and strong inner arches.

KYPHOSIS
Forward bending or curving of the spine. Extreme forms are known as Dowager's hump and humpback. Even minor forms contribute to back pain (cf. lordosis).

KYPHOTIC
Characterized by extreme forward curvature (cf. lordotic).

INTERCOSTAL MUSCLES
Muscles that run between the ribs, helping to form and move the chest wall.

L5-S1
The portion of the low back where the lumbar and sacral spines meet, specifically between the fifth lumbar vertebra and the first sacral vertebra.

LESSER TROCHANTER
See Trochanter, lesser.

LONGUS COLLI MUSCLE
A long muscle that twists and bends the neck forward.

LORDOSIS
Backward bending or arching of the spine, particularly in the lumbar area (cf. kyphosis).

LORDOTIC
Characterized by extreme backward curvature (cf. kyphotic).

LOW BACK
The lower portion of the spine, composed of five vertebra (L1-L5). Same as lumbar spine.

LUMBAR SPINE
The lower portion of the spine, composed of five vertebra (L1-L5) (cf. cervical spine, thoracic spine).

LUMBOSACRAL ARCH/ANGLE/CURVE
The natural arch of the low back, between the last lumbar vertebra and the sacrum (L5-S1).

MIDLINE GROOVE
A long, narrow furrow running vertically along the spine.

NEUTRAL SPINE
The state of the spine when it is neither overly flat nor overly curved, but held in a normal state of balanced tension.

OBLIQUE MUSCLES
Muscles at the side of the abdomen about at the level of the waist that compress the viscera and flex the thorax forward.

PECTORAL MUSCLES
The muscles of the chest: pectoralis major (which flexes, rotates, and adducts the arm), pectoralis minor (which raises ribs and draws down shoulder blades), and subclavius (which elevates first rib and draws clavicle down).

PELVIC RIM
See iliac crest.

PELVIC TILT, PELVIC TUCK
Two positions of the pelvis. A pelvic tilt moves the upper portion of the pelvis anterior to the lower portion. A slight pelvic tilt is desirable; an exaggerated pelvic tilt can lead to lordosis. A pelvic tuck moves the lower portion of the pelvis in line with, or even anterior to, the upper portion. An exaggeratged pelvic tuck can lead to kyphosis.

PRONATION OF FEET (FLAT FEET, FALLEN ARCHES)
A condition where the arch or instep of the foot collapses and approaches or comes in contact with the ground.

PSOAS MUSCLES
Two muscles of the lower spine: psoas major (which rotates the thighs and bends the spine) and psoas minor (which flexes the spine).

PUBO-COCCYGEAL MUSCLE (PC, KEGEL MUSCLE)
A hammock-like muscle, found in both sexes, that stretches from the pubic bone to the tail bone forming the floor of the pelvic cavity.

QUADRICEPS MUSCLE
A large muscle on the anterior surface of the thigh that extends the leg, and is composed of four smaller muscles: the rectus femoris, the vastus lateralis, the vastus medialis, and the vastus intermedius.

RECTUS ABDOMINUS MUSCLE
A paired muscle that runs vertically on each side of the abdomen from the pubis to the lower costal cartilages.

RETROVERSION
Inclining backward without bending (cf. anteversion).

RHOMBOID MUSCLES
Muscles that connect the inner borders of the scapula (shoulder blades) to the thoracic spine.

ROTATORES
Muscles of the back that rotate and extend the vertebral column.

SACRUM
The triangular bone that is located at the top of the pelvis and the base of the spine.

SITZ BONES
See ischial tuberosities.

SPINAL COMPRESSION
The act of applying an unusual amount of pressure on the spinal column, often resulting in pain due to damage to a spinal disc, fracture of a vertebra, or pressure on a nerve.

STERNUM
The long, flat bone in the middle of the rib cage. Also called the breastbone.

SWAY BACK
See lordosis.

THORACIC SPINE
The middle portion of the spine, composed of 12 vertebra (T1-T12) (cf. cervical spine, lumbar spine).

TIBIALIS ANTERIOR (SHIN SPLINT MUSCLE)
A muscle that runs from the outer lower leg to the inner foot. It acts to dorsiflex and invert the foot.

TRACTION
The process of pulling a limb, bone, or muscle group to align it or relieve pressure on it.

TRANSVERSE ARCH
See arches of the foot.

TRANSVERSUS MUSCLE
A flat muscle that forms the lateral and anterior walls of the abdominal cavity.

TRAPEZIUS MUSCLE
Muscle in the upper back that rotates the shoulder blades (scapula), and draws the head back and to the side.

TROCHANTER, LESSER
One of the bony outgrowths below the neck of the femur.

VERTEBRAL LEVEL
Any reference point along the vertebral column.

BIBLIOGRAPHY

(1) Volinn, E. The epidemiology of low back pain in the rest of the world: A review of surveys in low- and middle-income countries. Spine. 1997;22(15):1747-54.

(2) Fahrni WH. Conservative treatment of lumbar disc degeneration: our primary responsibility.

(3) Darmawan J, Valkenburg HA, Muirden KD, et al. Epidemiology of rheumatic diseases in rural and urban populations in Indonesia: World Health Organisation International League Against Rheumatism COPCORD study, stage 1, phase 2. Annals of Rheumatic Diseases. 1992;51:525-28.

(4) Darmawan J, Valkenburg HA, Muirden KD. The prevalence of soft tissue rheumatism. A WHO-ILAR COPCORD study. Rheumatology International. 1995; 15:121-24.

(5) Wigley RD, Zhang NZ, Zeng QY et al. Rheumatic diseases in China: ILAR-China study comparing the prevalence of rheumatic symptoms in northern and southern rural populations. J Rheumatol. 1994;21(8):1480-90.

(6) Dixon RA, Thompson JS. Base-line village health profiles in the E.Y.N rural health programme area of north-east Nigeria. African Journal of Medical Science. 1993;22:75-80.

(7) Anderson RT. An orthopedic ethnogoraphy in rural Nepal. Med Anthropol. 1984;8(1):46-59.

(8) Farooqi A, Gibson T. Prevalence of the major rheumatic discords in the adult population of North Pakistan. British Journal of Rheumatology. 1998;37:491-95.

(9) Chaiamnuay P, Daramwan J, Muirden KD, et al. Epidemiology of rheumatic disease in rural Thailand: a WHO-ILAR COPCORD Study. Journal of Rheumatology, 1998;25:7.

(10) World Health Organization and The Bone and Joint Decade, 2001.

(11) Lehrich JR, Katz JM, Sheon RP. "Approach to the diagnosis and evaluation of low back pain in adults"; UpToDate.com; April 2006.

(12) Deyo RA, Phillips WR. Low back pain. A primary care challenge. Spine. 1996;21(24):2826-32.

(13) Siambanes D, Martinez JW, Butler EW, et al. Influence of school backpacks on adolescent back pain. J Pediatr Orthop. 2004;24(2):211-17.

(14) Luo X, Pietrobon R, Sun SX, Liu GG, et al. Estimates and patterns of direct health care expenditures among individuals with back pain in the United States. Spine. 2004;29(1):79-86.

(15) Shelerud, RA. Epidemiology of occupational low back pain. Clin Occup Environ Med. 2006;5(3):501-28.

(16) Punnet L, Pruss-Ustun A, Nelson DI, et al. Estimating the global burden of low back pain attributable to combined occupational exposures. American Journal of Industrial Medicine. 2005.

(17) Hartvigsen J, Leboeuf-Yde C, Lings S, et al. Is sitting-while-at-work associated with low back pain? A systematic, critical literature review. Scand J Public Health 2000; 28(3):230-9.

(18) Lebouef-Yde DC. Body weight and low back pain: A systematic literature review of 56 journal articles reporting on 65 epidemiologic studies. Spine. 2000;25(2):226.

(19) Heliovaara M. Risk factors for low back pain and sciatica. Annals of Medicine. 1989;21(4):257-64.

(20) www.swissmasai.com

(21) MacGregor AJ, Andrew T, Sambrook PN et al. Structural, psychological, and genetic influences on low back and neck pain: A study of adult female twins. Arthritis Care and Research. 2004;51(2):160-7.

(22) Battie MC, Videman T. Lumbar disc degeneration: epidemiology and genetics. J Bone Joint Surg Am. 2006;88 Suppl 2:3-9

(23) Leboeuf-Yde C. Smoking and low back pain: a systematic literature review of 41 journal articles reporting 47 epidemiologic studies. Spine 1999; 24(14):1463-70.

(24) A special health report from Harvard Medical School: Low back pain: Healing your aching back. Ed: Jeffrey N. Katz. Boston:Harvard Health Publications, 2006.

(25) Harkness EF, Macfarlane GJ, Silman AJ, et al. Is musculoskeletal pain more common now than 40 years ago?: Two population-based cross-sectional studies. Rheumatology. 2005;44:890-95.

(26) White AH. The Posture Prescription: A Doctor's Rx for Eliminating Back, Muscle, and Joint Pain, Achieving Optimum Strength and Mobility, Living a Life of Fitness and Well-Being. Three Rivers Press, 2001.

(27) "Posture and back health: Paying attention to posture can help you look and feel better"; Harvard Women's Health Watch; August 2005:6-7.

(28) "Position yourself to stay well: The right body alignment can help you avoid falls and prevent muscle and joint pain"; Consumer Reports on Health; February 2006: 8-9.

(29) Jackson RP, McManus AC. Radiographic analysis of sagittal plane alignment and balance in standing volunteers and patients with low back pain matched for age, sex, and size: a prospective controlled clinical study. Spine. 1994;19(14):1611-18.

[30] Fahrni, W. Harry and Trueman, Gordon E. (1965): Comparative Radiological Study of the Spines of a Primitive Population with North Americans and Northern Europeans, The Journal of Bone and Joint Surgery, 47-B (3): 552.

[31] Fullenlove, T.M., and Williams, A.J. (1957): Comparative Roentgen Findings in Symptomatic and Asymptomatic Back. Radiology, 68, 572.

[32] Hult, L. (1954): The Munkfors Investigation. A study of the Frequency and Causes of the Stiff Neck-Brachialgia and Lumbago-Sciatica Syndromes. Acta Orthopaedica Scandinavica, Supplementum No. 16.

INDEX

A

Achilles tendon 190
arms
  numbness 35
  positions, lying on back 61
  positions, lying on side 105
  tingling 35

B

back, lying on 59
back pain 24
  cited causes 6
  fashion industry, influence of 15
  kinesthetic tradition, loss of 13
  real cause 10
  statistics 6, 11, 113
backrest
  car 51
  chair 38
back stretches, conventional
  35
beds 65
bending 152
  with knees 155
bones
  acetabulum 23, 171
  cervical spine 34, 123
  femur 157, 171, 179
  heel 145
  hip joints 171, 172
  hip socket 23, 171
  lumbar spine 50, 131, 163
  natural position of 22
  pubic 21
  rib cage 39, 84
  sitz bones (ischial tuberosities) 21,
    154, 162
  spine
    comparative illustrations 12
    ideal shape of 21
  thoracic spine 50, 163
breathing 23, 64, 72

C

car, healthy sitting in 43, 50
cautions
  bending activities 28
  bone spurs 206
  herniated disc 28, 73, 97, 206
  high impact activities 28
cervical pillows 66
cervical spine 34

chairs 38, 90
  backrest 38
  inadequate, modifying 49
circulation 23, 34, 35, 36, 48, 130, 131,
  172
corsets, external 124

D

discs
  bulging 153
  compressing 96, 113, 131, 155, 198
  damage 21
  decompressing 34, 114, 122
  herniated iii, 28, 153
  L5-S1 21, 73, 124

E

exercises
  abdominal muscles 197
  alphabet 201
  arches 211
  arm raise 200
  boat 203
  cycling 199
  eat the cloth 212
  gluteus medius 213
  grab the ball 212
  hamstrings 208, 209
  hip rotators 210
  inchworm 211
  leg lifts 201
  leg scissors 201
  leg slide 200
  neck muscles 207
  opposite arm/leg stretch 204
  paper clip 210
  pectoral muscles 205
  plank 202
  psoas 210
  rhomboid muscles 206
  rib anchor 198
  Samba 203
  side plank 202
  tibialis anterior 214
  trapezius muscles 206
  wall stretch 208
  warrior III 204

F

fashion industry, influence of 15
feet
  alignment 35, 142
  arches 142, 143, 145, 171, 172, 190

during pregnancy 146
going barefoot 146
insoles 146
pronation 136
shape of 46, 81, 135
floor, sitting on 91

G

Gokhale Method˙
  barriers to success 30
  how it works 17
  learning it 28
  results 18

H

height 34, 106
hunching 34, 49, 50, 96
hyperextension, knees 22

I

inner corset 112, 117, 118, 144, 153,
  162, 163, 190
insoles 146

K

kidney-bean shaped feet 81, 135
kinesthetic tradition, loss of 13

L

L'Institut d'Aplomb xvii
legs 137, 138
ligaments 22, 35, 146, 153, 155
lumbar cushions 50

M

mechanical advantage 164, 174, 192,
  198
muscles
  abdominal oblique 112, 114, 140
  abdominal transversus 114
  abductors (inner thigh) 186
  erector spinae 96, 114, 122, 154, 163,
    215
  external hip rotator 162
  gluteals 138, 170, 171, 172, 177, 181,
    190
  hamstring 21, 101, 154, 155, 158, 162,
    163, 179, 208, 209
  inner corset 112
  intercostal 122
  intrinsic back 112, 155
  Kegel (pubo-coccygeal) 21, 73

leg 170, 172, 190
longus colli 123, 124, 143, 144
psoas 62, 101, 171, 172, 175
quadriceps 175, 190
rectus abdominis 114, 215
rhomboid 49, 154, 155, 159
rotatores 123
tibialis anterior 135

N
neck
    alignment 34, 60, 103
    lengthening 44
Noelle Perez xvii

O
Olduvai Gorge 191
orthotics 146

P
pain and discomfort
    arthritis 10, 22, 130, 171, 172
    back pain 6
    bending 152
    bone spurs 22
    bunions 130
    carpal tunnel syndrome 34
    circulation 23
    cold feet 23, 97, 130
    disc damage 21
    dowager's hump 22, 153
    flat feet 145
    foot problems 22
    hip problems 23
    injuries, slow healing of 23
    knee problems 22
    ligaments 35, 130
    menisci, frayed 22
    organ prolapse 73
    osteopenia 22
    osteophytes 22
    osteoporosis 10, 22, 131, 172
    plantar fasciitis 22, 130
    Raynaud's Syndrome 23, 130
    repetitive stress injury 34
    sciatica iii, 10, 24
    sesamoid bone fractures 22
    shin splints 214
    urinary incontinence 73
    varicose veins 130
pillows 65, 103

posture
    anteverted pelvis 18, 20, 70, 71, 72,
        89, 130, 152, 171, 174
    buttock muscles 18
    chin position 18
    feet, angled outward 20, 142
    groin, angled 18, 130
    head position 18, 152
    healthy posture, elements of 18
    hinge at hip 153
    hunching 34, 76
    kyphosis 76, 153
    L5-S1 18
    line of vision, changed 89
    lordosis 76
    low back shape, assessing 76
    lumbo-sacral arch 18, 21, 97, 152, 198
    lying on side
        fetal position 96
        leg positions 108
        neutral spine 106, 107
        zig-zag shape 100
    lying on stomach 107
    neck position 35
    pelvic organs, affect on 21, 73
    pelvic position, assessing 75
    pelvis nested between legs 160
    retroverted (tucked) pelvis 20, 114,
        130, 175
    shoulder position 18, 152
    slumping 70
    spinal groove, midline 18, 77, 157,
        162
    spine, ideal shape of 21
    swaying 34, 76, 96, 122, 131
    torso shape 18
    weight over heels 20, 130, 142

R
rib anchor 84, 140, 198

S
Samba 191, 203
shoes 146
shoulder roll
    benefits of 34
    mechanism of 42
shoulders
    alignment 43, 60, 103, 143
    repositioning 49

spine
    comparative illustrations 12
    lengthening 34, 112, 122
success stories
    back injury 24
    back pain 25
    Ben Davidson 24
    Esther Gokhale xvii
    foot pain 172
    Gail Mahood 25
    Honor Rautmann 172
    Julie Dorsey 25
    kyphoscoliosis 125
    low back pain 24
    Milton Lozoff 25
    neck injury 24
    neck pain 25
    Paul Ehrlich 24
    sciatica 24, 25
    spinal stenosis 25
    Suzanne Hecker 25
swaying 34, 122, 131

T
traction 41, 47, 48, 51, 96
    benefits of 34, 56
    while sitting 34

W
walking on a line 186
    Laetoli duo 191
wedges 71, 80
    improvising 88

SUMMARY GUIDE

1. STRETCHSITTING

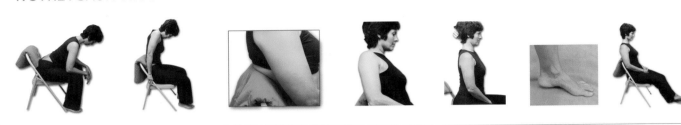

2. STRETCHLYING ON YOUR BACK

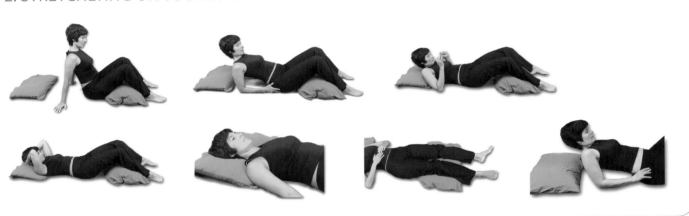

3. STACKSITTING

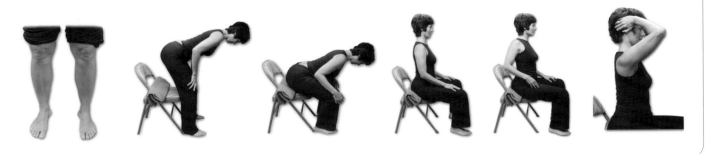

4. STRETCHLYING ON YOUR SIDE

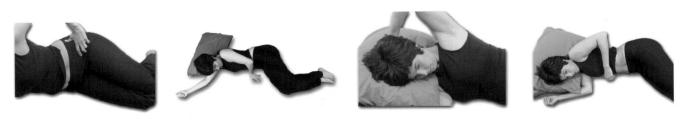

5. USING YOUR INNER CORSET

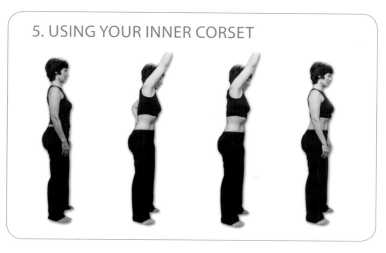

6. TALLSTANDING

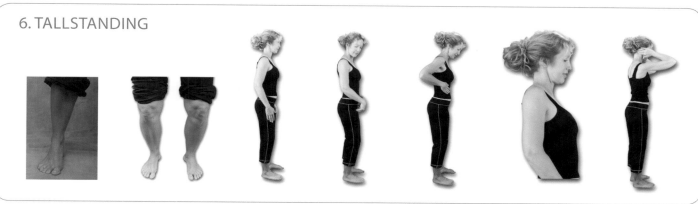

7. HIP-HINGING

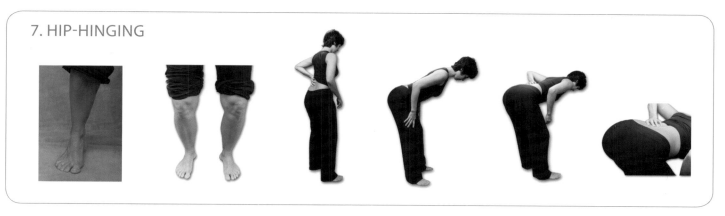

8. GLIDEWALKING

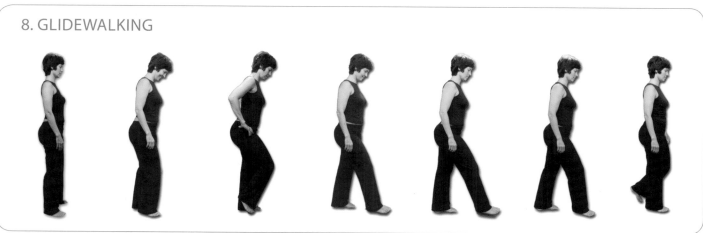

Further Offers for readers of
8 Steps to a Pain-Free Back

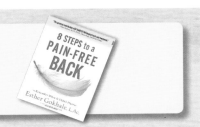

Gokhale Method Foundations Course

Nothing works as well as hands-on guidance from a qualified teacher! In six private or small group (eight people) classes offered worldwide, you can transform your structure and forever end back pain.

"I finally understand how my body is supposed to work! The content and quality of the course are unmatched. It is remarkable to undergo such a drastic change in so gentle a manner. This is a life-changing method."
- Eric Schoenfeld, Google, Mountain View, CA, Group GMF Alum

To register, visit **gokhalemethod.com**

Become a Gokhale Method Teacher

- Acquire an exciting new career in six months
- Begin changing people's lives immediately
- Help reduce the incidence of pain
- Transform your physical & mental well-being

Learn more at **gokhalemethod.com/teacher**

Stretchsit™ Cushion

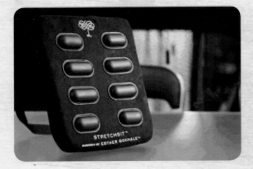

The Stretchsit cushion rejuvenates you by stretching your back and gently decompressing your spinal discs and nerves. It comes with an extension strap and can be used with almost any kind of chair.

Learn more at **gokhalemethod.com/stretchsit**

Gokhale Pain-Free™ Chair

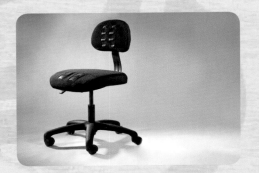

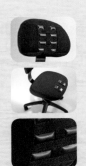

The Gokhale Pain-Free™ Chair celebrates the philosophy that sitting is a natural, healthy activity. Our chair facilitates stretchsitting and stacksitting, two techniques that transform sitting into a comfortable position and something that heals you rather than hurts you.

Learn more at **gokhalemethod.com/chair**

DVD - Back Pain: the Primal Posture™ Solution

Join Esther Gokhale as she addresses the root cause of most muscle and joint pain with healthy posture and movement techniques. Four real students are profiled as they successfully navigate degenerative disc disease, spinal arthritis, stenosis, back muscle spasms, sciatica, bunions, neck pain, shoulder pain and migraines.

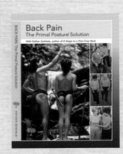

This DVD brings to life the techniques described in *8 Steps to a Pain-Free Back*. Special features include:

- Glidewalking
- Interview with Esther Gokhale
- Abdominal exercises

Order at **gokhalemethod.com/dvd** or on **Amazon.com**

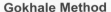
Gokhale Method

esthergokhale

Positive Stance™

Forum

www.gokhalemethod.com   **1-650-324-3244 • 1-888-557-6788**